"Make room on your bookshelf. Dr. Brenda Montecalvo's *Visual Secrets for School Success* is a treasure chest of insights and practical advice. Her "secrets" are a product of her personal and professional life. The story of how she came to them makes for fascinating and inspiring reading. What a gift to this generation of young learners and generations yet to come!"

—Adele Faber,
author of *How to Talk So Kids Will Listen
& Listen So Kids Will Talk*

"As a parent, I can speak to the change Dr. Montecalvo's pre-scribed vision therapy made in my son's life. My husband and I attributed certain behaviors of our then early school-aged son to age or clumsiness or inattentiveness. This was particularly true after taking our son to see an eye doctor and getting him the prescribed glasses. However, the issues continued. It wasn't until taking him to see Dr. Montecalvo that we discovered he had no depth perception, his prescription was incorrect, and his eyes were not working well together. This explained why he loved reading if we were reading to him--but was steadfastly reluctant to read on his own. As an educator, I am thankful for the succinct strategies this book provides for supporting our students who may be struggling. The book also helps us to consider seeking outside assistance when what we know how to do isn't enough."

—Jill Holland Beiser,
Principal, Curriculum Coordinator, Director,
Black River School District

"I found this book to be very well written, informative and easy to read. It makes an important contribution to the literature and will supply parents, teachers and other professions with critical information, which will help many children who are struggling to succeed in school and in life."

—Robert B. Sanet, OD, FCOVD,
Past President of COVD

"Visual Secrets is an excellent book for anyone interested in helping kids learn more efficiently, and to ultimately allow them the emotional freedom to excel in whatever life brings them. As an associate principal who has worked with at-risk students for 28 years, I can definitely say that these techniques will have a positive and long-lasting impact on students of all ages."

—Jim Heinke, Associate Principal,
West De Pere High School, De Pere, WI

"A must-read for parents whose child struggles in school. Dr. Montecalvo presents step-by-step instructions and engaging exercises that make schoolwork more manageable and even fun."

—Susan R. Barry, Ph.D.
Author of *Fixing My Gaze:
A Scientist's Journey Into Seeing In
Three Dimensions*

"Highly recommended to anyone interested in exploring how to save time by using vision more efficiently. Read *Visual Secrets for School Success* and change your student's life."

—Glen T. Steele, OD, FCOVD, FAAO,
Optometry Hall of Fame 2019 inductee,
and Professor of Pediatric Optometry at the
Southern College of Optometry

"A must for parents of school children. *Visual Secrets for School Success* is chock full of ideas to help make learning easier. Not only are Dr. Montecalvo's techniques effective, they are fun, too!"

—Robert Fox, OD, FCOVD, FCSO,
Past Chair of the COVD International Examination
and Certification Board

"Children don't come with instruction sheets, but this book will help you with strategies that can help your child perform better with less effort."

—Curt Baxstrom, OD, FCOVD, FNORA,
Past President of NORA

"Time is valuable, and *Visual Secrets for School Success* is certainly a worthwhile investment! Dr. Montecalvo's informative book will help students with writing, math, spelling and reading, giving them confidence and - best of all - free time!"

—Joanna Carter, OD, FCOVD,
Creator of VTODs on Facebook

"A down-to-earth practical guide for parents and teachers to help their children learn to use their vision more efficiently. End result: school work becomes easier, more fun and successful!"

—Lynn F. Hellerstein, OD, FCOVD, FAAO,
Award-winning author of *See It. Say It. Do It!*

"This book will be an important addition to my patient care. I have been effectively using many of the activities in this book for many years with my optometric vision therapy patients. It will be wonderful to have a resource to improve academic and study skills after we have corrected the functional vision problems!"

—Kellye Knueppel OD, FCOVD,
Wisconsin Optometrist of the Year

VISUAL SECRETS FOR SCHOOL SUCCESS

READ FASTER, WRITE BETTER, MASTER MATH AND SPELLING

DR. BRENDA MONTECALVO

Printed in the United States of America
Published by Author Academy Elite
P.O. Box 43, Powell, OH 43035

Identifiers

CCN: 2019938866
ISBN: 978-1-64085-650-9 (paperback)
ISBN: 978-1-64085-651-6 (hardback)
ISBN: 978-1-64085-652-3 (ebook)

Available in paperback, hardback, e-book, and audiobook.

Any internet addresses (websites, blogs, etc.) and telephone numbers printed in this book are offered as a resource. They are not intended in any way to be or imply an endorsement by Author Academy Elite, nor does Author Academy Elite vouch for the content of these sites and numbers for the life of this book.

Illustrations by Madilyn Heinke and Natalie Montecalvo, MS, OD

Disclaimer

The author and publisher of this book have used their best efforts in preparing the materials and activities described herein. The information in this book is for educational purposes only. It does not replace any medical advice by your optometrist or physician. The reader should regularly consult with a licensed optometrist for vision-related issues. The information provided herein is provided without any representations or warranties, be they expressed or implied. Mention of specific companies, organizations, or authorities does not imply endorsement by the author or publisher, nor does mention of specific companies, organizations, or authorities imply that they endorse this book, its author, or publisher. The author and publisher disclaim any liability for any medical outcomes or physical complications that may occur as a result of the application of methods suggested in this book.

Some names and identifying details in this book have been changed for confidentiality.

Dedication

This book is dedicated to Andrew, Clarice, and Natalie, who inspired me to gather the ideas shared here so we could spend more quality time together.

CONTENTS

Part III:
The Treasure: Time to Excel

ACKNOWLEDGMENTS

Twenty-five years ago, Dr. Ameil Franke heard my ideas about improving academic performance and said, "Brenda, you need to write a book." I have not forgotten that moment, and finally it is a reality. Thank you to Dr. Franke for believing in this book's potential.

Deepest gratitude and thanks go to my mentors, colleagues and friends that have challenged me, given me guidance, and made me think: Dr. Marilyn Heinke, Dr. John Streff, Dr. Baxter Swartwout, Dr. Robert and Linda Sanet, Dr. Al Sutton, Dr. William and Diana Ludlam, Dr. Donald Heiden, Dr. Donald Getz, Dr. Gerry Getman, Dr. Harold Haynes, Dr. Felisa Fernandez Lombardero, Dr. Cordula Stocker-Klug, Dr. Kellye Knueppel, Dr. Robert Fox, Dr. Brandon Begotka, Dr. John Pulaski, Dr. Valerie Frazer, Dr. Jeff Getzell, Dr. Mary VanHoy, Dr. Curt Baxstrom, Dr. Dean Streff, Dr. Carl Hillier, Dr. Lynn Hellerstein, Dr. Glen Steele, Dr. Glen Swartwout, Dr. Gary Busch, Dr. Rachael White, Dr. Michael Earley, and Dr. Susan Barry.

To my patients, who are also my teachers, thank you. From you I learn a little more each day. I appreciate your trust in my skills and in my ideas to help you reach your goals.

To the staff at Nova Vision Care, I am indebted to the entire team for your support. You are always there at a moment's notice to help and serve each other and our patients. Each day we change lives together; without your dedication this would not be possible. Thank you for your patience through this long book-writing process.

To Anthony Montecalvo, Dr. Kellye Knueppel, Megan Hook, Dr. Clarice Montecalvo, Dr. Natalie Montecalvo, and Laura Zeitner, I am so fortunate to have such dedicated editors. Your patience, guidance, and attention to detail have helped me create a remarkable finished product. Thank you Dr. Jamie Jacobs, Jennifer Buzecky, Charleen Heinke, Jim Heinke, Madilyn Heinke, Dr. Cathy Stern, and Dr. Joanna Carter for reading the draft manuscript and providing feedback.

To my strong, cheering, unstoppable mother, Dr. Marilyn Brenne Heinke, you are a beacon in my life both for your professional excellence and dedication to our family. Your belief in me and your guidance to the field of optometry have allowed me to continue the excellent care you gave your patients for 70 years. You were always looking for better ways to help people be more successful. I pray that I can continue to model your love for our profession and optometric vision therapy.

To my wonderful family, thank you for your love and support. Andrew, your hugs and kind, loving personality are such a joy to me and fills my heart. Clarice, your depth of caring and dedicated spirit to friends and family inspires me to see the beauty in everything. Natalie, your sensitivity and willingness to be supportive means the world to me. I know the three of you will always be there for me, no matter what.

To Anthony, my loving husband and the most important person in my life. You are my rock. You constantly help, guide, and inspire me. Without you I would not be who I am today. There are no words that can describe all that you mean to our family. Thank you so much for the many years of support, your excellent proofreading ability, and your coaching me to be better. I love you more than I can say or write. I am so blessed that God chose you for me. I love you.

Finally, I thank my Lord and Savior for all that He has sacrificed for me and for the many blessings He has given me. I strive each day to try to be a servant to others, as He taught us to be.

INTRODUCTION:
WHOSE KIDS ARE THEY?

On a blustery November day I peered out of my dining room window, spied the bright yellow school bus rounding the curve, and watched it approach our driveway. After the bus stopped with red lights flashing, the doors flung open and our three young children emerged. Smiles adorned their faces as they ran down the driveway with nearly empty backpacks slung over their shoulders. Seeing this filled my heart with love and joy, even though I had been a little anxious because that day was report card day.

Back in September, life had been drastically different. Earlier that summer, our family had moved from the suburbs to the country. Our new home was near a small town, which meant our children would encounter not just a new school system, but an entirely different academic program. At our previous home, our children were enrolled in a private Montessori school where they had enjoyed learning. It was acceptable to be a minute late. They never had to wear shoes in the classroom. They could learn at their own paces. They never had homework and were not given grades. Since our new home was too far from the nearest Montessori school, we enrolled them in the local public school. The school year started out with some stress, which included mounds of homework, having to wear shoes all day, and the fear of being given detention, not to mention a whole new set of potential friends.

Trying to figure out a new school system quite different from what we were used to had been tougher than I had anticipated, but we rose to the occasion. We made many adjustments to how the children approached completing all of their assignments. On Thursday of the second week of school, Andrew had a list of words in his homework folder. I asked him what he needed to do with them. His response was, "Nothing, Mom." I suggested he learn to spell them just in case there was a test. With a moderate amount of resistance, he agreed. Sure enough, the next day there was a test on the words. Being the new kid from a Montessori school, he was not accustomed to a weekly spelling test. The fifth grade class had a spelling test every Friday, and all the kids knew this except for Andrew.

Performance feedback was also different for our children. Clarice took her first timed math test in third grade. Even though she had been able to multiply and divide three-digit numbers at the Montessori school, she had never been timed. She received her first "F" and still remembers getting her test back and how it made her feel.

In first grade Natalie was taught to do math using her fingers. Even though she had learned addition and subtraction with math manipulatives and also how to do it in her head, the habit of using her fingers took years to break.

In addition, there were chapters to read, math problems to solve, and a variety of other assignments to complete. We spent most of every evening trying to get it all finished. Somehow, we squeezed in dinner and occasional sport practices. We were either running to a sporting event or doing homework. Needless to say, I was frustrated with our lack of family time. The year before, we'd had time to play games, talk, go for walks, and hang out with friends. Trying to get it all done without the breaks we were accustomed to was taking its toll, even in this short amount of time.

The pressures of school began to chip away at each of my kids' self-esteem. As an optometrist working with children who have learning-related vision difficulties, I had seen firsthand how difficult and stressful homework was for the families of struggling children. I taught many parents how to help their children succeed. My patients found success in their school performance after they completed an Optometric Vision Therapy program to improve their visual skills. I was able to help them learn to use their new visual skills for each of their school subjects, and I knew I had to do something for my kids before the stress caused permanent damage to how they felt about themselves.

Toward mid-September, I was ready to have my family back. I decided they were *my* kids after 3:00pm, not the school's, and I needed to come up with a better solution. Fortunately, as an optometrist specializing in Optometric Vision Therapy, I had many ideas at my disposal. To avoid being the shoemaker with shoeless children, I sat down and developed strategies for my kids so they would be more efficient at completing their assignments in school. I separated the various subjects of handwriting, spelling, composition, mathematics, and reading comprehension into simple-to-understand games for my children. These techniques allowed them to learn to use their visual skills efficiently. The human visual process gathers information and sends it to the brain more quickly than the other senses do, and using vision at its highest efficiency saves time. This allowed my kids to learn additional material or enjoy more free time. I refer to these techniques as *Visual Secrets for School Success.*

In a short period of time my kids learned how to become more efficient learners, get most of their homework done while in school, and still get great grades. I am pleased to say that throughout their elementary and high school years, my kids brought home very little homework. They had learned how to read faster, learn spelling words at a glance, and compute simple math problems in their heads. While other students spent more time completing in-class assignments, my kids completed their assignments quickly and then started their homework. These Visual Secrets ultimately enabled more school success and allowed them to participate in a variety of sports, spend time with their friends, and graduate at the tops of their classes. Today, each of them has completed post-graduate programs. Andrew, the eldest, has a master of science degree in engineering, and Clarice, our second child, is a medical doctor. Natalie, the youngest, is following in her grandmother's and mother's footsteps as an optometrist, and has also earned a master of science degree. Teaching Visual Secrets to them helped build a strong foundation for learning.

—◦◦◦—

For over twenty years I have taught hundreds of children *Visual Secrets for School Success,* which resulted in minimal homework and better grades. The ideas in this book work! With more efficient learning comes more free time and less stress, and children with reduced stress have better self-esteem.

My family discovered that the demands of nightly homework chipped away at our quality time together. Quality time improves self-esteem, thereby creating a better life. This is the ultimate goal for those completing the activities detailed in this book. I want students to enjoy learning, to take less time accomplishing learning activities, and to feel good about their ability to do so. By creating this positive learning environment, students will go on to achieve their goals with less stress and ultimately live more fulfilling lives.

PART I

THE TRAP: OVERLOADED WITH HOMEWORK

1

NO MORE HOMEWORK?

MORE TIME FOR FAMILY AND FRIENDS

Life is a one-time offer; use it well.

— Pranav Malhotra

Wouldn't it be wonderful if students could come home with no homework and great grades, happy to experience life to the fullest? Is the burden of school assignments undermining the motivation and confidence of struggling students? Shouldn't students have free time with their family and friends? The answer is yes! Here you will see how this can happen for students both young and old.

A NEW WAY

To create this ideal environment, students need help learning information efficiently and in a shorter amount of time. What if they could get their assignments done between classes, or at the end of class while others were still working? They would have so much more time to do what they want to do for fun. For over 25 years I have provided workshops in my office for patients, educators and healthcare professionals on how to develop and use visual skills to improve learning. My patients have realized much success in the areas of handwriting, spelling, composition, math and reading by incorporating the ideas in this book. This new way of learning builds a struggling student's motivation and confidence, and reduces his stress. The concepts discussed in *Visual Secrets for School Success* can help all students achieve more with little to no homework, while still achieving great grades.

Students should use their free time in the classroom to complete the assignments for each subject. When they return home, their time should be spent with family and friends. Imagine if you asked an employee to work hard all day, work through their lunch breaks, and take all unfinished work home. The overworked employee would become discouraged and look for another job. Students overwhelmed with academic demands cannot change classrooms like employees can change jobs. They have little or no say about their learning environment.

It is life-changing when students finish most of their work in the classroom and have less than 30 minutes of assignments to complete at home. Imagine how wonderful it would be for family evening life if they could relax and not worry about the demands of homework. A goal of *Visual Secrets for School Success* is to regain quality family time. The ideas discussed will help the parent guide the student to become more efficient at learning, and achieve higher than expected results in the areas of handwriting, spelling, composition, math and reading.

COACHING

Be prepared to take on a coaching role rather than a parental role. Telling instead of asking is defeating, and coaching will help motivate struggling students and build their confidence.

ASK QUESTIONS INSTEAD OF TELLING THE STUDENT HOW TO DISCOVER THE RIGHT ANSWER.

Ask your student questions, instead of telling him the answer, so he can discover the correct answer. Always use positive statements. Showing the student what he did correctly is more helpful than always pointing out the mistakes. For example, when learning to spell the word "reptile", if your student spells it "reptil" you should say, "You have five of the six letters correct" instead of saying, "You spelled it wrong." Help the student self-evaluate so he can carry over that skill to the times when there are no coaches to help him.

In my experience I've seen struggling students talk back to their parents and not allow them to help. When learning Visual Secrets, the student needs to treat his parent as if he is a coach. You may need to remind him that sports coaches don't hear phrases like, *I can't*, *I don't want to*, or *I don't want to try that* from the players.

Ethan thought he was stupid.

Ethan's parents brought him to our office hoping to find answers to why he was struggling in school. Ethan had passed all of his visual screenings because they only tested his 20/20 eyesight, which gave his parents a false sense of security that his eyes were fine. The comprehensive optometric evaluation performed at our office, however, determined that his eyes did not track easily which caused him to lose his place when reading. He had focusing problems that made copying the blackboard difficult for him. His eye teaming skills caused a slight doubling during reading when he was tired. He showed difficulty with laterality concepts which related to his reversing "b and d, p and q". He also had no ability to make a picture in his mind of the words he read, so he had to sound them out every time he encountered the same word.

When I explained to Ethan that he was very smart but his eyes were not helping him perform at a high level, his lip began to quiver and a tear rolled down his cheek. He said, "I just thought I was too stupid to learn." My heart broke and I knew I would be able to help Ethan and change his life.

Ethan's vision problems were resolved upon completion of an optometric vision therapy program. He then had to learn how to use his newly developed visual skills. Using *Visual Secrets for School Success*, his parents and he began tackling one subject at a time until all of his subjects were easy to perform without effort.

Ethan went on to become an "A" student and, more importantly, to enjoy learning. His parents commented at one of his annual evaluations that he loved to read and always had a book in his hand.

Do not do the Visual Secrets activities with the student's siblings present. Sibling competition can be negative, especially when the student who needs the help has a more difficult time with the activities.

WHAT TO EXPECT

The following chapters take you, step-by-step, through the process of developing and using specific visual skills for the variety of subjects taught in school. You will learn to determine if your child has well-developed visual skills, how to establish those skills that aren't well developed, and then how to coach him on using those skills for maximum efficiency. This will save time for everyone. We only have a finite amount of time while on this earth. The older we get, the more evident this fact becomes. My goal is to help students optimize their time so they can be more efficient and effective for a lifetime, and go on to achieve their dreams.

Get ready to learn how to improve handwriting, because it sets a good impression for a lifetime. Learning cursive writing increases activity in the same areas of the brain in which reading comprehension is processed. In this book you will discover how to improve spelling, which is an important skill that can make or break a future job interview. Handwriting and spelling, while not dependent on one's level of intelligence, are significantly important in creating a good impression. Poor penmanship or spelling lowers the opinion of others about your abilities, and often lowers their expectations. This can affect job promotions, being chosen for a position on a committee, or how others perceive your ability to do a job.

This book also provides information on how to develop the ability to write excellent compositions. This skill is critical when putting together a scholarship application, applying for college, writing a thank-you note, drafting a business proposal, or publishing your first book.

Mathematics can be easy for all, not just the exceptionally high-achieving students. Math is all about measuring space in many different ways, which is a completely visual concept. By helping students *see* what math represents, we can make it easier for them to understand it. The chapter on mathematics gives strategies on how to easily and enjoyably learn math facts. Math facts are simply memorization. Most kids don't like flashcards, and this book will teach math skills using different activities. Knowing math facts helps get tougher math assignments completed correctly in a shorter period of time.

Chapter 8 is about reading comprehension. While likely one of the most difficult skills to improve, it is the most important—not only for academic success, but also for building self-esteem and fulfilling lifetime goals. Enjoyment of reading opens up so many more opportunities for lifetime learning, personal development, and career advancement. The activities discussed in this chapter will help students enjoy reading and improve comprehension.

Chapters 9 through 11 show the importance of developing visual skills for a lifetime of high-quality learning. They discuss the significance of every second, and how it is critical to not waste a moment. These chapters guide the student in developing organizational and management skills to effectively implement the *Visual Secrets for School Success*.

How to Proceed

Visual Secrets for School Success is packed with great ideas that will improve a student's learning abilities. To begin the process of using these Visual Secrets, ask the student which subject he would like to improve first. Often this will be his best subject, which is fine. Improving a skill that the student enjoys will be quicker and create a more positive environment than working on a more difficult one.

After reading the ideas contained in this book, students and their coaches may feel overwhelmed. To manage this, work on only one subject at a time and don't do more than 30 minutes at a time. Each chapter of this book is broken down into sections:

Section	Application
Components and Concepts	The distinct parts of each subject area
Building Skills	Development of the student's ability to use the components and concepts
Practice	Activities for building automaticity and avoiding use of splinter skills
Troubleshooting	Identifying roadblocks that interfere with a student's ability to develop their skills, and proposing solutions to overcome them

The following example shows one week of activities. An entire 12-week program is provided in Appendix #6. Use this program as a guide, and tailor it to your student's individual needs.

Week 1	Time	Chapter	Spelling Activities
Day 1	2 hours	2	Setting up Study Space
Day 2	10 min.	5	Stacking Cups
Day 2	15 min.	5	MONTECALVO Spelling Technique for 10 words
Day 3-5	10 min.	5	Parquetry Block Memory
Day 3-5	15 min.	5	MONTECALVO Spelling Technique for 10 words
Day 6	20 min.	5	Practice Spelling Test
Day 7			Enjoy Family Time and Play Time

If your student has mastered the ability to use the components and concepts, you can skip the Building Skills section and perform the Practice activities until they are easy and automatic for him.

If your student struggles with the Building Skills section, it is fine to increase the number of days suggested in the example above until he masters the skills. Remember to vary the activities to avoid boredom.

SUMMARY

Using *Visual Secrets for School Success* is a new way to learn. This book teaches techniques for handwriting, spelling, composition, math, and reading comprehension, along with organization and management skills. Parents act as coaches. Students who are able to complete assignments in class or during study hall will have little to no homework and less stress. They will be happier because they will have more time for family, friends and extracurricular activities. Their improved well-being will have a positive effect on their approach to school assignments and other requirements. They will become more motivated and confident about their abilities. The students will excel and exceed expectations, which will boost their self-esteem. Use the ideas discussed in *Visual Secrets for School Success* and watch your student transform.

2

STOP STUDENTS' STRUGGLES!
SET THE STAGE FOR SCHOOL SUCCESS

*Whether you think you can or think
you can't, you are right.*

— Henry Ford

A six-year-old ballerina was on stage for her first recital. During her performance, she had a wonderful time—even though she ran into the ballerina to her right and turned the wrong direction several times. On the way home, her parents raved at how well she had done and how hard she had worked to learn the dance steps. They predicted that she would one day be a prima ballerina.

A six-year-old baseball player was up to bat for his first game of t-ball. The first swing was a strike. The second was a hit. He ran as fast as he could to third base, not to first base. The crowd chuckled a little but cheered loudly. On the way home, his parents called him their little slugger and said one day he would be a famous baseball player.

The little girl and the little boy were in class together and had completed their first writing assignment. When they got their papers back, there were red marks all over them. There were spelling errors and grammar errors, and their handwriting was difficult to read. When the children got home, their parents frowned and said that they needed to try harder. Why, at six years of age, do we expect adult performance on school assignments but not in any other areas of students' lives? Before entering school, students have not been exposed to much failure. They've played with friends, had fun in preschool, and been the apples of their parents' eyes. Upon entering school, the unsuccessful students go from a positive world to daily criticism. Family life goes from harmonious to stressed.

BEFORE BEGINNING ON THE ROAD TO CHANGE HOW OUR STUDENTS LEARN, IT IS IMPORTANT TO SET THE STAGE FOR OPTIMAL LEARNING.

Visual Secrets for School Success helps to reduce these struggles. Before beginning on the road to change how our students learn, it is important to set the stage for optimal learning. Think about all of your senses. Each one affects how you perform, feel, and think. The senses of sight, smell, touch, taste, and hearing should all be considered when creating the perfect study area in your home. This chapter reviews how to design this study area for your student. Include your student when selecting some of the items listed below. However the coach will need to overrule the selection when it would result in a study space that creates a negative attitude that interferes with the eye-brain process.

The following is a list of important considerations to provide the student the best opportunity to learn:

1. Lighting

2. Ergonomically correct furniture

3. Music

4. Color

5. Temperature

6. Hydration

7. Diet

8. Vision breaks and exercise

9. Aroma

10. Digital device use

11. Sleep

12. Attitude/positive coaching

LIGHTING

Today there is a push for more fluorescent lighting in school and at home to save money and be more environmentally friendly. Although these considerations are important, we should also consider how the fluorescent light is affecting our physiological systems and eye-brain processing.[1] Clinically, my patients with autism, stroke, and brain injury have more severe visual stress symptoms when under fluorescent light than under incandescent light.

The healthiest light is sunlight or candlelight, followed in order by full-spectrum incandescent lighting, halogen light, light emitting diode (LED), and compact fluorescent light (CFL). Fluorescent is the most common form of lighting in schools; however, it is the most difficult under which to study and can be very disruptive to a reader's eyes and visual process. To reduce exposure to fluorescent light in the workplace or school, a brimmed hat or visor can be prescribed.

This is a list of some of the possible side effects of fluorescent lights.[2]

1. Eye strain

2. Eye pain or inflammation

3. Blurred or impaired vision

4. Difficulty reading or focusing

5. Headache or migraine attacks

6. Vertigo or dizziness

7. Lightheadedness

8. Shortness of breath

9. Nausea

10. Lethargy

11. Anxiety

12. Feelings of depression

13. Disrupted sleep

Other effects of fluorescent lighting include:

1. neurotoxicity from mercury inside the bulb [3]

2. radiation emission; there are certain types of radiation that can be harmful [3]

3. high amounts of blue light that affect sleep [3]

4. potential increase in overactivity [4]

5. more difficulty for the brain to process information [5,6]

6. muscle tension [3]

A study done in a first-grade classroom showed that dynamic light had a positive effect on oral reading fluency.[7] Dynamic light is defined as the change in the quality of illumination and color temperature of the light based on the activity being performed. Dynamic light will change depending on the student's needs throughout the day. For example: one type of lighting should be used for quiet time, and a different type used for times when the student needs to be more alert.

ERGONOMIC FURNITURE

Darrell Boyd Harmon, PhD specialized in studying the process of growth and development in the school child, with emphasis on the psycho-physiological and visually-centered aspects of learning, together with the effect of the environment on those processes. Dr. Harmon published several works regarding improvement of ergonomic conditions in the classroom. He determined that improved ergonomics would in turn develop better handwriting, cognition, and performance.[8]

Comfort is invaluable when studying and learning new skills. In order to achieve this comfort, the study area selected should contain the correct table height and chair height for the student. If a student is uncomfortable while doing the activities listed in this book, it will be difficult for him to pay attention and concentrate. A chair that is the correct height will allow the student to place his feet flat on the floor with the knees bent at a 90-degree angle. Dangling feet do not allow for proper position and this interferes with the eye-brain process. Proper posture allows for better body tonicity and for good circulation so oxygen can get to the brain. Good posture helps with alertness, concentration, and comfort.

The table height should allow the student to write or read the materials on the table at a distance known as the Harmon Distance. In Illustration #1, "E" to "b" is the distance from the elbow to the knuckles. This is equal to the distance from "a" to "b", which is the distance the eyes should be from the reading or writing material. If the table is too high, the eyes will be too close to the material to be comfortable. If the table height is too low, the student will hunch over the work, which affects circulation and back comfort.

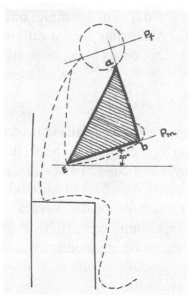

Illustration #1: Proper Seat and Desk Position, Journal of
Optometry History, vol. 49 #4 (2018)

MUSIC

Music influences attitude and behavior. Research has shown
that music can create a pleasurable mood, and can change
how the brain processes information. In addition, it can have
a positive effect on attention while completing a task. One
study found that music helps the brain to pay attention.[9] The
type of music chosen also influenced brain processing and
improved cognitive function when the music improved the
student's emotional state.[10] Studying while listening to music
can be beneficial because music, memory, and emotions are
strongly linked.[11]

Self-selected, quiet background music may improve your
student's ability to focus. Optometric Vision Therapy encour-
ages multi-sensory tasking, and students who complete an
OVT program develop the ability to be less distracted by
background noises. This makes it possible for music to enhance

performance. Note: A student who has difficulty with sensory integration may find music too distracting.

COLOR

Blue is a background enhancer, while red is a figure stimulator. If the background is blue and you put a red purse in the center, the eyes will automatically be drawn to the red purse because central eyesight is more attracted to red.[12] Too much red, however, will over-stimulate. Use a red pencil and point to the part of the assignment needing attention. Don't make the whole assignment red by using red letters or using red paper.

Color can influence mood and emotions. Considerable research has been conducted on using color in sales and marketing, resulting in this understanding. Colors can influence how much time is spent in a store, the level of pleasant feelings while shopping, the number of purchases, and the image of the store. For store displays, red tends to be more negative while blue tends to be more positive.[13] Use these ideas to set the stage in the study area to create the appropriate emotions for learning. Some students will need to relax and de-stress while others may need to wake up a bit. Students are individuals, so coaches must watch, listen, and learn what is best for their students.

A color overlay is a sheet of transparent acetate that is placed over reading material to change eye comfort when reading. It will not harm the visual system to use an overlay if the student feels it helps with attention. Research on the effectiveness of color overlays, however, has been inconclusive.

Colored lenses over the eyes have more influence on the eye-brain process than using a color overlay. If you use colored lenses, do not use them for more than 20 minutes because too much of one color may result in extreme mood changes toward either anxiety or depression.

The color of the desktop surface should also be considered. A green or blue desktop may be beneficial and less distracting.

Avoid black, gray, or too much orange and red. The following is a list of possible effects of different colors.

Color	Effect
Green	Restful for eyes and reduces eyestrain
Orange	Energizes and increases brain activity
Yellow	Joy
Blue	Relaxation and stability
Black	Aggression
Blue/green	Calm, hopeful, reduces anxiety
Grey	Passive, lack of energy

Again, how a student reacts to the various colors is specific for that individual. The effects in the table above are generalities. If you select a color and it is unpleasant or causes stress, try a different color. Some optometrists who provide vision therapy are also trained in light therapy to treat visual conditions that interfere with learning. This is a highly specialized area known as optometric syntonic phototherapy. These practitioners are usually members of the College of Syntonic Optometry and can help you determine the best color for your individual student. For more information see Appendix #1.

AROMA

A pleasant aroma can create a positive mindset and behavior, and memories are often attached to certain aromas. Pleasant odors can influence how long a shopper will stay in a store. For example, the scent of bread in a bakery can influence the shopper to increase his purchase.[14] The smell of chocolate in a bookstore has a positive effect on cookbook sales.[15] The wrong smell, however, can cause a violent reaction such as nausea.

There is a close neurological connection between smell and memory because the emotional brain is more closely linked to the smell receptors than to any other sense. Find out what aroma is pleasing to your student. You can use certain aromas to direct certain behaviors, but too much of one aroma may become negative. For me, too much of a pleasant room air freshener becomes overpowering and is no longer enjoyable. From personal experience, less is best. A faint background smell will be more positive than a strong one, and it will be tolerated for a longer period of time.

The following is a list of possible effects of aromas.

Aroma	Effect
Vanilla	Reduces anxiety
Coffee	Creates alertness
Lemon	Helps with concentration
Rosemary	Helps memory
Peppermint	Benefits clear thinking
Frankincense	Improves problem solving
Cinnamon	Reduces mental fatigue
Lavender	Increases accuracy

TEMPERATURE

A study from Cornell University found that reducing the room temperature to 68 degrees Fahrenheit or colder resulted in employees making 44 percent more errors.[16] The study determined the optimal room temperature was 77 degrees Fahrenheit.

> A STUDY FROM CORNELL UNIVERSITY FOUND THAT REDUCING THE ROOM TEMPERATURE TO 68 DEGREES FAHRENHEIT OR COLDER RESULTED IN EMPLOYEES MAKING 44 PERCENT MORE ERRORS.

The study stated that when a person is cold, energy is diverted to keep warm and takes away from the ability to concentrate. The study also noted that being warmer also made people happier. When dining out with my family, I always bring a sweater and a blanket. If the restaurant is cold, I will not be able to enjoy the time with my family or my meal.

If the study area is difficult to heat without making the entire home too warm, you can use a blanket or small room heater during study times. Have a thermometer nearby to keep track of the temperature. This will serve two purposes:

1. Keeping the room at the correct temperature

2. Teaching the student how to read temperature, and the difference between Fahrenheit and Celsius

HYDRATION

Our bodies are comprised of 60 percent water, and water is a conductor of all of the electrical impulses that occur within our bodies. There are millions of impulses occurring each second in our eye-brain process. When a student becomes dehydrated, the eye-brain process will not be optimum. It has been shown that hydrated children have better memory.[17] Headaches, fatigue, and lightheadedness are early signs of dehydration. To check a student's level of hydration at home, pinch the skin on the back of the hand, hold for a few seconds, then release. If the skin is sluggish to return to normal, he is dehydrated. It is important to encourage adequate water intake.

DIET

The Centers for Disease Control and Prevention reported that a well-balanced diet will provide the necessary nutrients to stabilize energy levels that in turn create optimal alertness, increase focus, and improve overall academic performance.[18]

Foods that can help boost memory:

- Leafy green vegetables

- Salmon and other cold-water fish

- Berries and dark-skinned fruits

- Coffee and chocolate

- Extra virgin olive oil

- Cold-pressed virgin coconut oil

What do these items have in common? They contain nutrients that have a direct impact on the eye-brain process. When food is high in omega 3, lutein and zeaxanthin, there is improved cognitive ability. Besides being good for the eye-brain process, these foods are also noted to be good for overall health. High-sugar and high-carbohydrate snacks do not create the best eye-brain process possible. In moderation, they are not too disruptive. In large quantities, however, they can have a huge negative impact on the eye-brain process.[18] Some negative effects may include drowsiness or hypoactivity, sometimes referred to as "brain fog."

VISION BREAKS

Everyone, both students and coaches, needs a break. Each student is unique and the amount of time working between breaks will vary; younger students need more frequent breaks. The breaks need to involve movement. Standing up and walking to the kitchen to get a drink of water is an example of a good break. Walking to the living room and sitting on the sofa to watch TV is not recommended because the eye-brain process is not getting a rest. Every fifteen minutes the student should look out the window at something, and think about what he is observing. This gives the visual process a quick escape, which reduces stress. Getting the "feeling" sense involved is even better. Seeing a robin looking for worms and hoping that she finds enough to feed all of her babies is an example of involving the "feeling" sense.

The physical breaks should be every 30 to 45 minutes for younger students, and every hour for older students. If a student has a significant attention problem, more frequent breaks are recommended.

The break should only last 5 to 10 minutes. So, select an activity that is not too involved.

Here are some ideas for breaks:

- Ten jumping jacks

- Washing the dishes

- Shooting a few basketballs

- Playing with the cat or dog

- Feeding the cat or dog

Downtime is an opportunity for the brain to make sense of what it has recently learned. Rest allows the student to release unresolved tension and to turn reflection from the external to the internal world.[19]

> DOWNTIME IS AN OPPORTUNITY FOR THE BRAIN TO MAKE SENSE OF WHAT IT HAS RECENTLY LEARNED.

EXERCISE

Regular exercise is good for both the coach and for the student. Take a walk together. Walk the dog. Go biking or take an exercise class together. Hike in the woods or go horseback riding. This will establish a lifetime habit of taking time to exercise. A fit body has a better chance to stay focused during study times and fit students feel better about themselves.

DIGITAL DEVICES

Reduce time spent on digital devices that aren't required for school. Digital addiction is real and can hurt a student's ability to turn the written word into meaning. Lengthy, passive viewing of digital devices will cause the brain to be dependent on passive stimulation. This happens because all of the visual imagery is already provided for the eye-brain process. Creative, interactive eye-brain processing is minimal when viewing digital devices. Reading, however, is an active process because the eye and brain must convert a bunch of black letters into visual meaning or imagery. When the content is complicated, it is easier for the brain to use active processing. Too much passive learning makes the eye-brain process "lazy", and there is little experience or interest in converting information because it has always been provided. The more difficult reading is for a student, the more important it is to reduce digital device use.

> DIGITAL ADDICTION IS REAL AND CAN HURT A STUDENT'S ABILITY TO TURN THE WRITTEN WORD INTO MEANING.

Quality of sleep can be negatively influenced by overuse of digital devices such as cell phones, tablets, laptop or desktop computers, and television. Avoid watching any digital device within two hours of sleeping. Play a board game, read, or go for a walk instead.[20]

ATTITUDE

Be a motivating coach to help create a positive attitude within your student. If you do not receive the correct response or answer, you did not ask the right question. Help the student discover how to do an activity, rather than telling how it is done. When the student is frustrated, don't try to make suggestions to improve the situation. Instead, repeat the problem as stated by the student, and wait for or encourage the student to come up with a solution. Ask, "What do you think you should do about . . ."

Create the most positive environment you can. It can be extremely frustrating when a student faces challenges when trying to learn. When both coach and student are frustrated, take a break and re-group. Do something you enjoy together.

Try to avoid using digital devices during the break. Some suggestions: take a walk, play a board or card game, shoot a few hoops, or bake a box cake. There are many possibilities. Sit down with your student during a non-study time and make a list of his or her favorite things to do. Explain that the list can be very creative. Also, explain that no digital device activities are allowed on the list.

Be sure to do the techniques for Visual Secrets in Chapters 4 through 8 at least five days each week to establish a positive pattern of learning.

SUMMARY

Creating a positive learning environment for optimal success during study times involves many considerations. Making a special space that is enjoyable will help your student stay focused when the learning material is difficult. Remember, each student is an individual with specific likes and dislikes. Involving your student in creating the special study space will ensure that he feels relaxed and good about his or her study area.

3

WHAT IS VISION?

20/20 EYESIGHT IS NOT ENOUGH TO SUCCEED IN SCHOOL

When vision works well it guides and leads;
when it does not, it interferes.

— John Streff, OD

VISION VERSUS EYESIGHT

Eighty percent of sensory input is visual. We use vision to know our environment and where we are within it. Vision is the only sense that requires muscular/motor action, such as when throwing a ball. The senses of smell, taste, hearing, and touch are passive. Vision does not occur in the eyes, it occurs in the brain.

Regular eye exams check the eye organ, but not always the eye-brain (or visual) process. One can have 20/20 eyesight and still have a vision problem that makes learning difficult, thus students' vision problems are usually missed because they are not related to visual acuity. It is the eye-brain process that can get mixed up. There are at least twenty visual skills important for learning that are not directly dependent upon having "perfect" 20/20 eyesight at distance. If these visual skills are poorly developed, it can be harder to reach one's fullest potential.

Problems in the classroom can be caused by an undiagnosed learning-related vision difficulty. Since one in four children has a vision problem that interferes with learning, it is not surprising that students who struggle in school often have vision problems that have been missed.[21] The types of vision difficulties that affect learning are rarely visual acuity, or 20/20 eyesight, issues. The most common learning-related vision problems involve eye tracking, near point focusing, eye teaming, and visual-perceptual (or eye-brain) processing. These types of vision problems increase with fatigue, excessive near work, and increased use of digital devices.

Vision problems are often hidden. They can develop over time, or they can be acquired from many types of injuries to the brain. Unaddressed, they can result in disability, problems with daily living activities, fatigue, confusion, or anxiety because the visual input to the brain doesn't match the other sensory inputs or the actual physical world.[22]

More than 80 percent of information learned in the classroom is dependent on vision.[23] Many students with learning-related vision problems, however, pass the eyesight screening given by the school nurse or at the physician's office.

THERE ARE AT LEAST TWENTY VISUAL SKILLS IMPORTANT TO LEARNING THAT ARE NOT DIRECTLY DEPENDENT UPON "PERFECT" 20/20 EYESIGHT AT DISTANCE.

This may be confusing because we've been told that 20/20 eyesight is the "be-all, end-all" when it comes to good vision. Most binocular vision disorders and major eye problems in the early stages of disease, however, do not cause blurred or painful vision. Examples of binocular vision disorders include eye tracking problems and focusing problems. Examples of eye diseases include glaucoma, diabetic retinopathy, macular degeneration, and cataracts. Therefore, one cannot depend on pain-free eyes and clear eyesight to determine one's eye health, or how well the eyes work together. Instead, one should get a comprehensive eye examination by a highly trained eye doctor who understands all parts of eye health and vision issues.

THE VISUAL SYSTEM

The human visual system is directly linked to the brain by a complicated, intricate process that influences everything a person does. Vision is involved in all activities required for school, sports, hobbies, and work. It is critical that one's visual system works as well as possible to permit optimal performance.

Dr. Darrell Groman has specialized in Optometric Vision Therapy (OVT) for twenty-five years. He says that in school we have always been taught about the human eye as if there is only one eye. See Illustration #2. What is missing in this picture when we are learning about the human eye? The other eye is missing! Humans have two eyes, and they are the only moveable parts of the brain.

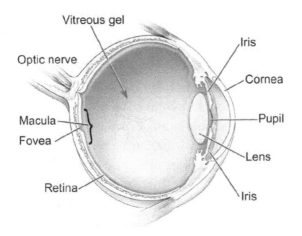

Illustration #2: The Human Eye

However, human eye anatomy continues to be taught the same old way, with the entrenched notion that 20/20 eyesight is all that is required for normal and perfect vision. The concept of "The Human Eye", singular, is taught beginning in 5th grade—and then continues to be taught in the fields of medicine, nursing, psychiatry, and other professions interested in the study of the developing human being, despite the fact human beings have two eyes.

A camera analogy is often used when explaining how the eyes work. This is a poor analogy. The only similarity between a camera and the eye is that in both cases light enters through an aperture or pupil; after that, the process is dramatically different. A camera has an aperture and the eye has a pupil. Both change based on how much light is available. Cameras make pictures. The eyes send information to the brain to organize the information to create meaning so it can be understood. The eye and the visual process are only like a camera if it is capturing a movie, and you include the photographer and the director of the movie. In order to see and understand what is viewed, the light from both eyes must be coordinated before the brain knows what to do with it. This coordination of light from the two eyes is much easier if the image is clear, single, judged to be the same size and shape, and accurately located. This process involves all parts of both eyes, their pathways that go to all areas of the brain, previous visual experiences, and an entire body of neurological feedback processes that fine-tune and better understand what is being seen.

Not everyone can point both eyes to the same place at the same time. There are many who have double (or overlapping) vision, which cannot be diagnosed when examining only one eye at a time. In addition, focus and attention become difficult when there is blur instead of clarity, double vision instead of single vision, high visual effort instead of effortless vision, or uncomfortable instead of comfortable vision. What is also poorly understood is that vision intertwines with behavior.

WOW, THIS SOUNDS COMPLICATED!

Yes, it is complicated and intricate, and it takes an optometrist many years of post-graduate education to understand the entire eye-brain process. Upon graduation, only some eye doctors continue to learn about these processes. Others stay more focused on eye health, which mostly involves the eyeball and clear 20/20 eyesight. In reality, 20/20 eyesight represents about one two-hundredth of the entire visual processing system.

There are non-optometrists with minimal information and little training that assess and treat visual conditions. They understand much less about eyes and vision than optometrists do, and falsely believe they can do no harm. Many individuals check their own eyes by determining how clear everything looks to them. When this happens many vision and eye health problems will go undiagnosed and untreated. Everyone should have a comprehensive eye health and vision evaluation each year by an optometrist or ophthalmologist to be sure every part of the eye and vision process works correctly and is healthy. One of our most precious gifts is sight. Keep it working well for a lifetime with regular visits to your eye doctor.

To get a better understanding of the big picture it helps to know what visual skills are involved with the visual process.

VISUAL SKILLS

There are a whole bunch of visual skills. You do not need to understand each visual skill, but your eye doctor does. A clean bill of health and a full visual assessment from a specialized eye doctor ensures your student will have vision problems identified and addressed. Then your student will be able to effectively use the *Visual Secrets for School Success* discussed in Chapters 4 through 8.

These specialized eye doctors will evaluate more than eyesight (20/20 visual acuity) and eye health. They are well-trained to assess visual-motor and visual thinking skills important for learning, and they provide Optometric Vision Therapy.

Visual skills critical for optimal performance are discussed in upcoming chapters. Each subject of handwriting, spelling, composition, math, and reading requires a unique set of visual skills. Combined, there are many visual skills important for overall learning. Thus, there are many areas of vision that can help or interfere with performance. See Appendix #2 for a list of visual skills important for learning.

HOW DO I KNOW WHICH EYE DOCTOR TO VISIT?

Only certain types of eye doctors are educated and highly trained to evaluate and treat vision problems that interfere with learning. These types of eye doctors (officially called "optometrists") specialize in Optometric Vision Therapy (OVT). Other terms that may be used to define these types of eye doctors are behavioral, functional, or developmental optometrists. These eye doctors have specialized training, and usually belong to organizations such as the College of Optometrists in Vision Development, the Optometric Extension Program, the Neuro-Optometric Rehabilitation Association, or the College of Syntonic Optometry. See Appendix #1 for a list of these organizations. Each year, optometrists earn over 100 hours of continuing education related to vision and learning. Be sure to ask the optometrist specific questions to help you assess his ability to provide the service your student needs. See Appendix #3 for questions to ask. If your eye doctor can answer "yes" to these questions, rest assured that your student will receive all necessary tests, assessments, and treatment recommendations to achieve optimal visual skills for success in all school subjects. These optometrists can also help guide you through the activities discussed in Chapters 4 through 8.

CHOOSING THE DOCTOR

WHY DO I NEED A SPECIAL EYE DOCTOR FOR AN EYE EXAM?

A student's level of intelligence is less critical to learning than knowing how to use certain skills efficiently. Any student with a normal level of intelligence should be able to have legible handwriting, correctly spell all words on a spelling test, remember mathematical concepts, write an interesting story, and enjoy reading. When there is a vision problem, these skills are not easily acquired. Before you try the *Visual Secrets for School Success* activities, it is critical to get a complete, comprehensive eye health and vision evaluation by an optometrist who understands how vision relates to school performance.

OPTOMETRIC EYE HEALTH AND VISION EVALUATION

Often, when students have developed new visual skills, they do not automatically start using them for learning. This book will help bridge the gap so that students can realize high levels of academic success when using these ideas. Therefore, this book is not intended to be a substitute for an optometric examination or Optometric Vision Therapy. It is designed for students who have developed the visual skills required to perform academic tasks in handwriting, spelling, composition, math, and reading. If your student has an annual comprehensive eye health and vision examination and your optometrist has determined all visual skills are properly developed, you will find the suggestions for each academic skill very useful. When a specific visual skill has not yet been developed, a program of Optometric Vision Therapy under the direction of an optometrist to build that visual skill may be needed for the student to be successful in school. See Appendix #4 for a checklist your optometrist can use to ensure proper tests are conducted to assess the visual skills necessary to improve success in handwriting, spelling, composition, math, and reading.

Remember, not all eye exams are exactly the same. When assessing visual skills important for learning, an evaluation is needed that can determine how well specific visual skills are developed. High-quality eye health and vision examinations typically take longer, and may consist of more than one visit.

> THIS BOOK IS NOT INTENDED TO BE A SUBSTITUTE FOR AN OPTOMETRIC EXAMINATION OR OPTOMETRIC VISION THERAPY. IT IS DESIGNED FOR STUDENTS WHO HAVE DEVELOPED THE VISUAL SKILLS REQUIRED TO PERFORM ACADEMIC TASKS IN HANDWRITING, SPELLING, COMPOSITION, MATH, AND READING.

WHAT EXACTLY IS OPTOMETRIC VISION THERAPY?

Optometric Vision Therapy (OVT) is a prescribed training and therapy program to develop, restore, improve, and/or correct visual skills that are interfering with performance at school, on the job or on the playing field. OVT retrains the eye-brain system to make more efficient use of how the eyes process visual information.

Vision is commonly thought of as a static system, but it is actually an active process. The utilization of vision is learned. OVT is the most effective way to learn how to use your vision. "An infant isn't born with an adult-like visual system; he or she must learn how to use it. Everyone learns differently and at a different pace; some need guidance and others do not." (Brandon Begotka, OD). Optometrist Dr. Vicky Vandervort says, "Optometric vision therapy is like speech therapy. There is nothing wrong with the tongue that says 'eth' instead of 'ess' just like there is nothing wrong with the eyeball that cannot send the right information to the brain."

Another way to understand OVT is through the computer analogy by optometrists Drs. Jennifer Ceonzo and Moshe Roth. They state,

"We see with our brains through our eyes. OVT is creating efficient software for the eye-brain process. Using vision to complete tasks is like using a computer and printer to type a letter. When you keep seeing a mistake on the printout, where is the problem? Might be a faulty keyboard (eye muscles and eyeballs), possibly a printer problem (hands, feet, fine motor) or the hard drive (eye-brain coordinating signals). OVT works on keyboard and hard drive problems. Eyes are like the mouse and keyboard of a computer. They are the most important input devices to get information into the computer. The brain is the computer processor. OVT enables the computer to use the software efficiently and enables a student to efficiently process more information, perceive, apply what is learned and arrive at new ideas and cognitions. OVT allows for better outputs like the computer monitor, printer or speakers. OVT helps students process better and improves the output devices (eye movements, eye/hand coordination, eye/body coordination)."

OVT not only addresses the ease of alignment of our two eyes, it also helps foster critical visual thinking and visual processing. This helps students have a better sense and understanding of who, what, when, where, and why. When the visual process works efficiently, students do not exhibit as many uncontrolled eye, hand and body movements. An example would be a student reaching for a glass of water. When the visual process tells the hand where to reach, his hand easily connects to the glass and lifts it. When the visual system misjudges where the glass is, it is easier to knock over the glass and spill the contents on the table. Uniquely designed therapeutic performance lenses and prisms will assist the students in the exploration of their world. These special lenses can enhance performance in academic and athletic endeavors in life, and your optometrist will be able to determine if your student will benefit from these lenses.

What is OVT?	What does OVT use?	What is the goal of OVT?
- A program of vision procedures performed under a doctor's supervision - Individualized to fit the visual needs of patients - In-office visits, once-or-twice-weekly sessions of 30 to 60 minutes, sometimes with homework	- Therapeutic lenses - Prisms - Filters - Occluders or patches - Timed electronic targets - Balance boards - Tools for specific activities	- Help patients develop or improve fundamental visual skills and abilities - Improve visual comfort, ease, and efficiency - Change how patients process or interpret visual information

This diagram is located at www.COVD.org

SUMMARY

Learning difficulties can involve an undiagnosed learning-related vision problem. The most common learning-related vision problems involve visual tracking, near focusing, eye teaming, visual-perceptual processing, or eye-brain processing. These types of vision problems increase with fatigue, excessive near work, and increased use of digital devices. Optometric Vision Therapy is a prescribed program that is the most effective way to learn how to use your vision successfully. Finding the right eye doctor will ensure proper assessment and treatment so your student has the best, most developed visual skills possible to be successful at using *Visual Secrets for School Success*.

PART II

THE TECHNIQUE: VISUAL SECRETS FOR LEARNING

4

VISUAL SECRETS FOR HANDWRITING

HANDWRITING AND FIRST IMPRESSIONS LAST A LIFETIME

In all the ways we express ourselves non-verbally nothing is quite as personal as our handwriting.

— Betty Edwards

Does a teacher initially regard a student with poor handwriting as academically inferior until proven otherwise? Does an employer disregard sloppy or illegible job applications? How might poor handwriting affect job promotions? What about applying for credit or loans? One day, when your student applies for a job, he or she will be asked to complete some paperwork just prior to the interview. If the handwriting used to fill out the paperwork is sloppy, then the interviewer may have a negative first impression of the applicant, even before the interview begins. On the first day of school, if a student turns in a paper with nice, neat handwriting, the new teacher will have a more positive impression of his abilities than if the writing on the paper was sloppy. Good handwriting can give a little extra edge for achieving better grades or one day getting called for an important interview.

When my kids switched from the Montessori school to public school I knew they would be graded on handwriting. My fifth-grade son Andrew had many poor handwriting habits, and his penmanship looked like that of a child in kindergarten. I worked with him for about two weeks to help him change the poor habits. By the middle of fifth grade his teacher held up his paper and exclaimed it was the best handwriting of the class.

In schools today, less emphasis is being placed on the importance of cursive handwriting. This is occurring mostly because of the thought that computers have replaced the need to have good handwriting. Also, teaching cursive is being dropped by many schools to allow time to teach the new Common Core standards. New research provides strong evidence that cursive handwriting should be kept in school curricula. The new evidence suggests there are strong links between handwriting and overall educational development of reading and writing.[24] Learning cursive helps develop areas in the brain important for recognizing words, which has a positive effect on reading.

Research points to the fact that children learn to read more quickly and are able to generate ideas and retain information more efficiently after acquiring good penmanship skills. Recent evidence also shows there is a unique neurocircuit created when we write in cursive. This neurocircuit creates a special way of improving word recognition. Three areas of the brain important for reading are stimulated when we write words. Finally, children with better handwriting have more neural activations in areas associated with memory, which activates creative thinking.[25] The evidence clearly points to the importance of handwriting skills for

> RESEARCH POINTS TO THE FACT THAT CHILDREN LEARN TO READ MORE QUICKLY AND ARE ABLE TO GENERATE IDEAS AND RETAIN INFORMATION MORE EFFICIENTLY AFTER ACQUIRING GOOD PENMANSHIP SKILLS.

student learning. If a school has decided to stop teaching handwriting skills, parents must help children learn to write in cursive correctly. This chapter on handwriting provides ideas on how to help make handwriting a joy instead of a chore.

FIRST IMPRESSIONS

While it is true that no good data exist linking intelligence and handwriting, many people have a pre-conceived notion that poor handwriting is equivalent to low intelligence. For this reason it is still very important to have nice handwriting. Attractive handwriting gives a great first impression because those viewing the handwriting will automatically think better of one's ability to be neat and well-organized. It is quite common for individuals who observe poor handwriting to judge a person's intelligence and neatness based on their handwriting. When writing is difficult, composition can suffer, too. This is because the student writes shorter sentences and smaller words just so they don't have to write as much. Poor handwriting ability can affect performance in school and other aspects of life.

See Illustration #3. Read both entries. Get a sense of your impressions of the writers of the two paragraphs. If the first paragraph is a first-grader and the second an executive, there will be no difficulty recognizing that. If the first paragraph is the executive and the second an unsuccessful student, that information may not match with your initial impression. If the first one is a doctor, that may match your impression because doctors are one of the few professions that are excused for poor handwriting. These mismatches occur because our brains constantly make decisions about what we observe.

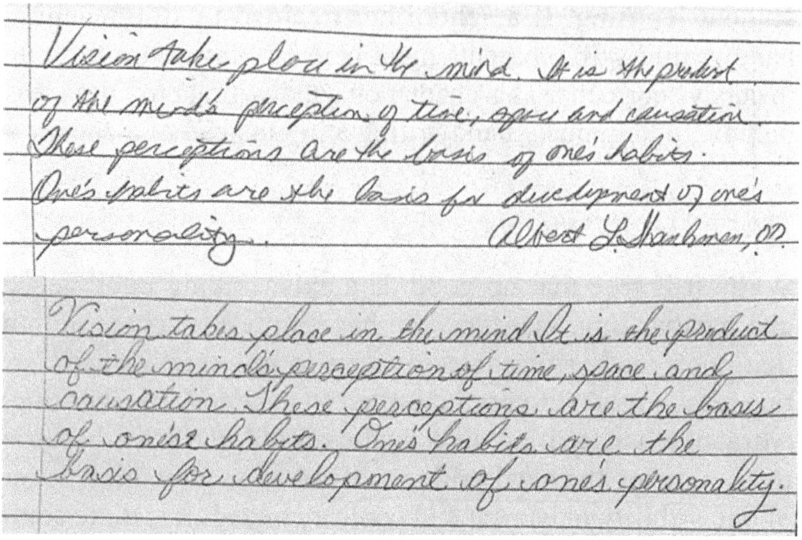

Illustration #3: Two Examples of Handwriting

WHY IS HANDWRITING SO DIFFICULT FOR MANY STUDENTS?

One reason for poor handwriting is that children are required to write before they are developmentally ready to perform the skill with ease. Learning to write before developing the fine motor skills needed for good penmanship results in using bad habits in order to accomplish the task. The ability to write easily and effortlessly requires good fine motor control and is usually developmentally present by the time girls reach nine years of age and boys reach ten years of age. In order to complete required writing assignments prior to these ages, many children must adopt habits that interfere with good penmanship. These habits can last a lifetime, so when a child is developmentally ready to write well, the bad habits interfere with the ability to display good handwriting skills. This chapter on handwriting will teach how to retrain and develop good fine motor skills for solid penmanship and how to coach students so they can break habits that interfere with neat handwriting.

Specific visual skills are needed to complete the handwriting activities in this chapter. If a student has problems in one or more of the visual skills listed or it is unclear if these are well developed, schedule an appointment with an optometrist who specializes in Optometric Vision Therapy for an assessment and treatment of these skills. See Chapter 3 for information about finding the best optometrist for your student.

VISUAL SKILLS FOR HANDWRITING

The visual skills important for good handwriting include:

Visual Skill	Definition
Smooth Pursuits	Maintaining fixation on an object while the eyes are following it in any position of gaze
Accommodation	The ability to keep an image in focus when viewed up close
Single vision	Seeing one object when looking at it with both eyes
Peripheral Vision	The ability to subconsciously be aware of what is not being looked at. This may also be referred to as side vision
Hand-Eye/ Fine Motor Coordination	The ability to coordinate the hand with the eyes

Pursuits: When a student has problems with pursuits, he will not be able to keep the tip of the pencil on the correct line while writing.

Accommodation: Focus is important for seeing which line the pencil tip should be touching when writing. The entire writing assignment requires constant focusing.

Single vision: Double vision, or seeing two images when there should be one, makes it very difficult to consistently place the letters. When the line or pencil tip is double while writing, the letters can end up in the wrong place.

Peripheral Vision: This type of vision is important for knowing where the pencil is going and for writing straight lines on the page with good spacing. The eyes should guide the hand; if peripheral vision is compressed it is difficult for the eyes to anticipate where the pencil should go. Holding one's breath while writing or being overly stressed can create temporarily constricted peripheral vision.

Hand-Eye Coordination: When the eyes misjudge where objects are, then the hand controlling the pencil may overshoot or undershoot the line on the paper. Poor coordination is evident when handwriting is sloppy and unorganized.

TIME NEEDED

You only need ten to fifteen minutes each day to improve handwriting. Use part of the time to practice learning three letters, and the other part doing activities to improve hand manipulation and flexibility. After about two weeks, the new hand and body positioning for creating good handwriting will become more automatic. Once automaticity occurs, the practice time usually is reduced to about five minutes.

COACHING

Students need a coach, and for many children this is usually one of their parents. As discussed in Chapter 1, it is very important to remember the coach-student relationship. Don't "tell"—instead, ask questions when directing the student to fix or improve on performance. Use positive encouragement and statements so the student discovers how to correct areas that are not quite right. The coach's job is tough because he or she needs to be able to keep track of about fourteen different skills at one time and to encourage the student when corrections in position, pencil grip, and penmanship need to be made.

It is critical for students to look upon the coach as a coach and not as a parent. Think of it this way: on a sports team, the coach may ask players to change something to improve a skill. The player doesn't resist, and he does his best to do what the coach asks. Talking back to the coach, crying, or resisting suggestions might get the player benched, and then he won't get to play. The same expectations apply to coaching *Visual Secrets for School Success*. Developing positive behavior is best achieved with positive coaching. Coaches need to point out the good skills observed, and ask questions to help students discover how to change to get better. An example of positive coaching is asking, "Johnny, which two fingers are supposed to pinch the pencil?" versus saying, "Johnny, you are holding the pencil wrong." Positive coaching is critical to achieving the highest level of skills in the shortest time. The book *How To Talk So Kids Will Listen & Listen So Kids Will Talk* by Adele Faber and Elaine Mazlish is a resource for more ideas on how to achieve a positive environment for optimal success.[26]

John was frustrated with handwriting.

Although a bright child, he had extreme difficulty putting his ideas on paper due to his inability to write legibly. This led to poor grades in any subject that involved writing. John had learned to write when he was too young and had many habits that interfered with legible penmanship. He had difficulty managing a writing utensil and used a fist grip. He had a hunched-over posture and his nose was usually five inches from the paper. Working for about 10 minutes a night with his mom as a coach, he began to change his habits after just two weeks. He excitedly reported that he got a B+ on a writing assignment and the teacher had noted his paper was neat and readable.

MATERIALS NEEDED

Once the student's visual system has the appropriate visual skills needed for great handwriting, he or she will be ready to gather the items needed to create the best environment possible for top-notch handwriting.

- Special wide-lined paper with dashed centerline
- Pencil
- Chair so feet can be flat on the floor
- Table so eyes can be 16" from tabletop
- Slanted work surface (20 degrees)
- Highlighter
- 8" x 11" paper
- Hard clay
- Baton
- Deck of playing cards
- Bright non-fluorescent lighting

COMPONENTS OF HANDWRITING

1. The Desk and Chair

An old wooden school desk, with an adjustable seat and adjustable desk surface slanted at 20 degrees, provides correct body positioning. Dr. Darrell Boyd Harmon's research shows how critical the desk and seat are for optimal learning in the classroom.[27] This

DR. DARRELL BOYD HARMON'S RESEARCH SHOWS HOW CRITICAL THE DESK AND SEAT ARE FOR OPTIMAL LEARNING IN THE CLASSROOM.

position can also be created at any table by using a raised chair and propping the student's feet with a box. See Illustration #1 in Chapter 1 for correct sitting posture.

Once the table and chair height are correct, ensure that the top of the table is slanted 20 degrees. Alternatively, place a slanted surface on top of the table that is at 20 degrees. Appendix #5 provides resources to find slanted work surfaces. Another option is a three-inch, three-ring binder, which has a slant close to 20 degrees.

2. Body Position

The feet need to be flat on the floor with the knees bent at a 90-degree angle. If this is not possible, increase or decrease the size of the box used. Another idea is to use a stack of books on which to set the feet. The student's back must be straight without leaning on the back of the chair. The only body parts touching a surface should be the bottoms of each foot and the student's bottom toward the edge of the chair. This creates a tripod effect. The non-dominant hand's palm holds the paper, and the dominant hand holds the pencil properly and rests softly on the paper. The head and body should always be centered with the paper. There should be no head tilt or body shifted to one side. The distance from the eyes to the paper must be equal to the distance from the knuckles to the elbow. This is called Harmon's Distance.[27]

3. Proper Paper

The paper needed for the exercise is the type that is used in kindergarten, with wide lines and a dashed line in between the solid ones. You can find this type at school supply stores or online, or you can create your own. I prefer the ones that have portrait versus landscape orientation. See Illustration #4 for an example of the type of paper needed.

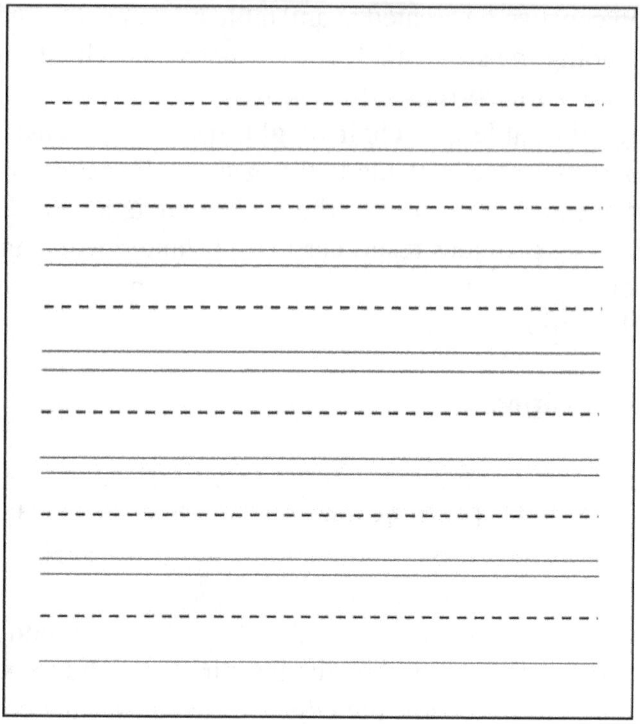

Illustration #4: Lined Dashed Paper

4. Pencil and Grip

Use a standard No. 2 pencil. With a permanent marker, draw a line around the pencil about one inch from the pencil tip. See Illustration #5. This line will be used to position the fingers so the tip will not be obstructed from view while writing. The goal is for all students to be able to write well with or without adding a writing aid or rubber pencil grip. These types of aids can feel quite comfortable if one needs to write for a long time, but for building this skill we do not use the rubber grips. They can be added, if desired, once penmanship is mastered. After mastering the Visual Secrets needed for good penmanship, the student will be able to pick up any writing utensil at any time and use it to create beautiful handwritten materials.

Pinch the pencil just above the marked line with the pointer finger and the thumb. Rest the pencil gently on the middle finger. See Illustration #5. Many times, students learn handwriting before their fingers are ready to grip properly and naturally. As a result, they develop an improper grip that interferes significantly with good handwriting. It will take lots of positive coaching to help change a poor grip to the correct one. This is critical, though, to achieve proper placement of letters and effortless penmanship.

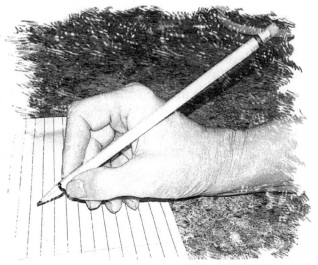

Illustration #5: Proper grip with line on pencil.

5. Breathing

Breathing is important because lack of oxygen decreases quality of performance. All Air Force pilots undergo training in a ground-based device that replicates the reduced oxygen that exists at high altitudes. The purpose of this training is for the pilots to detect their specific symptoms of lack of oxygen and to take corrective action if it happens while flying. When my husband Anthony, an Air Force F-16 pilot, was fulfilling this periodic training requirement he experienced what happens to one's vision when there is a lack of oxygen. One of the first signs of reduced oxygen can be tunnel vision, which occurs because the blood vessels furthest from the central vision must travel farther to provide oxygen to surrounding tissue. These vessels are often the first affected by decreased oxygen levels, thus halting vision processing. Holding one's breath to perform a task can result in temporary tunnel vision, which affects performance. The coach should monitor the student's natural, regular breathing while the student performs the hand-writing tasks.

6. Soft Touch

How often does a pencil tip break right after sharpening it in the sharpener? Why does this occur? The pencil breaks because the student uses an improper grip. When using the wrong fingers to grip a writing utensil, the writer has to push hard to manipulate the pencil, gets sore fingers, and breaks the tip. So, while participating in these handwriting activities, the student must write with a "soft touch." This means the mark on the paper is very light, not dark. I refer to this as "feather writing," which implies soft, light touch.

When I was in school I used my thumb and third finger to hold the pencil. I always broke the tip after sharpening my pencil because I held it too tightly and pressed too hard. This created a huge bump on my third finger. When I was in college I decided to change how I held the pencil. It took a while to change my habit, but eventually it felt natural to hold it correctly and the bump finally went away. My hand stopped hurting when I wrote and I no longer broke my pencil tips.

7. Eyes Lead the Hand

Some students often grip the pencil so close to the tip that their eyes cannot see where the pencil is going. The student is then writing blindly, with no regard to letter placement on the line. Thus it is critical that the pencil is gripped far enough from the tip so the eyes can see the point of the pencil and the line on the paper. This is why I suggest drawing a black line on the pencil: to guide the fingers to not get too close to the tip. If you sharpen the pencil, you will need to redraw the line so it is approximately one inch from the tip of the pencil.

Where are the eyes looking while writing occurs? Many incorrectly watch the point or tip of the pencil. The eyes should not be fixated on the tip of the pencil while writing. They should look ahead to the place the pencil tip is going. The job of the eyes is to guide and lead the hand holding the pencil. This will ensure the pencil tip is accurately placed.

Look at a cursive lowercase *a*. When beginning to write the letter, the pencil tip is placed at the bottom line. The eyes should be fixed on the dashed line, ahead of the pencil tip. That is where the mark is to go. The eyes move ahead of the pencil tip to guide it, so it can be placed correctly on the paper as the letter is written. If the eyes stray, the letter does not end up positioned correctly between the bottom line and dashed line.

Try writing your name while looking only at the tip of the pencil. Then, try writing your name looking ahead of the tip. Notice how much easier it is to place the letters properly when looking ahead of the tip of the pencil. The coach can observe the student's eyes to determine if they are keeping fixed ahead of the pencil tip by placing a mirror on the table next to the paper and watching the reflection of the student's eyes in the mirror. Coaches should ask the student to self-assess letter placement. Self-assessment is done with a highlighter, where the student highlights any part of the letter that is not correctly placed. The student should highlight lines that go over the line or are short of the line.

8. Up and Over

This part of the penmanship activity involves noting how the letters are formed. When the hand is tired and writing is difficult, the student takes shortcuts and only moves the fingers up and down instead of making large round motions with the arm and wrist. This creates penmanship that has many pointy-topped letters. See Illustration #6. Practicing with full arm movements and making large round clockwise and counterclockwise circles should be a precursor to cursive writing. I remember making lots of these large circles in first and second grade to get ready for cursive writing. Many times, this exercise is skipped to save time and the student does not develop correct hand motions to create nicely formed letters. While writing the letters, ask the student to make round letters with an up and over type of motion.

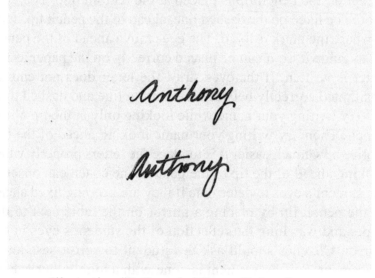

Illustration #6: Rounded Versus Pointy Letters

BUILDING HANDWRITING SKILLS

The fingers need to be ready to write. This is a developed skill, and various activities will help increase the neural connections between eyes, fingers, hands, and brain. The less you use fine motor activities with all of your fingers, the less efficient the brain is in performing handwriting activities. The more you do activities that require precise fine motor control, the easier good penmanship is to learn.

During one of my handwriting workshops a harpist performed every one of these activities without any effort. Her daily hours of harp practice gave her more experience watching her fingers manipulate the strings than the average person.

> THE LESS YOU USE FINE MOTOR ACTIVITIES WITH ALL OF YOUR FINGERS, THE LESS EFFICIENT THE BRAIN IS IN PERFORMING HANDWRITING ACTIVITIES.

In order for students to improve penmanship, they first need to participate in several activities that improve fine motor control and eye-hand coordination. Scientists have noted that professional musicians, who use more fine motor skills than non-musicians, have a larger array of neural connections in the motor, auditory and visual-spatial areas of the brain.[28] The message here is that the more you purposefully use your eyes with your hands, the better you develop control of your hands and fingers. The following activities are provided to help develop better finger-hand-eye coordination. This, in turn, will make penmanship activities much easier to perform well.

Note: Some students have extreme difficulty performing any of these activities. If this is the case ask your optometrist to recommend an assessment with an occupational therapist that specializes in developing fine motor control.

1. Paper Crunch

Material: 8" x 11" white paper

Procedure:

Step 1: Take one piece of 8" x 11" paper and fold it in half so the size of the paper is 8" x 5.5". Pinch the fold with the fingernail to make the fold more complete.

Step 2: Tear along the fold. It is important to show the student how to tear a piece of paper in half without using scissors so it rips only along the fold. This is accomplished by placing the non-dominant hand on the paper with the thumb or pointer finger at the part of the fold that is being torn. The dominant hand moves down the paper, keeping tension on the part being torn.

Step 3: After the paper is torn in half, hold each piece of paper in each hand, and hold the hands above the head. The arms and hands do not touch any part of the body.

Step 4: Crunch the paper in each hand so that the fist covers the entire piece into a small ball of paper. Do not let the elbow, or any part of the arm touch the body while crunching the paper.

Step 5: Now, keeping hands in the air, un-crunch the ball of paper in each hand and return it to its original size.

Note: Remember, do not touch anything but the paper while crunching or un-crunching. If you look at your hand while doing this activity it will be easier to perform crunching. A more advanced procedure is to do it without looking at the hands.

After teaching this workshop for years, it amazes me that very few students are taught how to tear a piece of paper in half on the fold.

2. Finger Lift

Material: Flat surface

Procedure:

Step 1: Place the student's hands palm-down on a table. Without touching the student's fingers, the coach points to one finger and asks student to raise it off the table without moving the other fingers. Repeat with each finger.

Step 2: The coach points to the pointer finger of both hands and has student raise them at the same time, without moving the other fingers.

Step 3: Repeat with thumbs and middle, ring, and pinky fingers.

Step 4: Next the coach points to two different fingers (for example, right pointer and left ring finger). The student should raise their fingers at the same time without moving the other fingers. Repeat with different finger combinations.

Step 5: Next, indicate three fingers to be raised, and repeat. Indicate four fingers, and repeat.

3. Paper Tear

Materials:

- A piece of paper
- Highlighter marker

Procedure:

Step 1: With the highlighter, draw a five-inch vertical line starting at the top edge of the paper, halfway between the left and right sides of the paper. The mark should be about one quarter inch thick, and fairly straight.

Step 2: At the location of the vertical line, the student grasps the top edge of the paper using the pointer finger and thumb of both hands in a pinch configuration.

Step 3: The student slowly rips the paper along the vertical mark so there is an equal amount of highlighter on each side of the torn pieces.

Note: Do not use other fingers—only the pointer and thumb. To increase difficulty, make the mark more irregular with curves and sharp turns. To decrease difficulty, make the mark fatter and straighter.

4. Clay Finger Roll

Material: Hard clay

Procedure:

Step 1: Take a small amount of clay, about a quarter of a teaspoon. The student rolls the clay between the dominant hand pointer finger and the dominant hand thumb into a perfect, small ball.

Step 2: Repeat with thumb and middle finger, then with thumb and ring finger, then with thumb and pinky. To increase difficulty, use the non-dominant hand instead. To further increase difficulty, complete task with both hands at the same time.

5. Baton Twirl

Material: Baton

Procedure:

Step 1: The student places the baton in the dominant hand and twirls it between thumb, pointer, middle, ring, and pinky finger, then back from pinky to ring to middle to pointer to thumb.

Step 2: Repeat with non-dominant hand. Then try using a baton in each hand.

Students really enjoy this activity; they are all eager to try it when it is demonstrated at workshops.

6. Card Shuffle

Material: Deck of playing cards

Procedure:

Step 1: The student splits the deck of cards in half using only one hand. This is very difficult for small hands. To shuffle the cards, put one half of the split deck in each hand. Weave the halves together by placing the thumb on one end of the deck, pointer finger bent in middle of the deck, and the rest of fingers holding the other end of the deck.

Step 2: To back-shuffle, make a bridge with hands around cards. For this, the thumbs are on top.

There are several online videos on how to shuffle cards. If the student's hands are too small, use fewer cards or smaller sized cards.

GETTING STARTED

Remember, you only need ten to fifteen minutes each day to improve handwriting. The good news is anyone at any age can improve his or her handwriting. Don't forget to be the coach.

PRACTICE

Plan to work on handwriting no more than ten to fifteen minutes each night. At each session, have the student do one activity to get the fingers ready to write. Then have him practice learning how to write three letters. Start with the first three letters of the alphabet. For the second session, choose the next three letters, and so on. Do this every night until all of the letters of the alphabet are learned.

At each session, encourage correct positioning of the three letters on the lined paper (Illustration #4). Note: If the student is still printing letters instead of writing cursive, have the student print the three letters with equal space in between the letters.

When the student has learned to correctly place and space the three letters, have him take a marker and highlight where the letters are not touching the correct parts of the top, middle, and bottom lines. If there are highlighted areas, ask the student to write all of the learned letters once again until there are fewer corrections.

Once this is accomplished, have the student connect the three cursive letters that he learned this session. Have the student check proper letter position with the highlighter. If the student can write the three letters and there is no need to highlight any parts of the letters, then the activity for that evening is complete.

After about two weeks of writing the alphabet from A to Z, the student will begin to notice the activity getting easier, and that it takes only a few minutes to accomplish. This is called *automaticity,* which means little thought or effort is required to accomplish the task.

Automaticity is important for all of the activities in this book. It helps ensure that the skills being developed will transfer to academic performance. An example of automaticity is learning to drive a car with a manual transmission. The steps (releasing the gas pedal, pressing the clutch petal, moving the stick shift to the correct gear, releasing the clutch petal, pressing on the gas pedal at the appropriate time) need to be in the correct order. Once the process becomes effortless or automatic, it can be repeated without conscious thought.

> AUTOMATICITY IS IMPORTANT FOR ALL OF THE ACTIVITIES IN THIS BOOK. IT HELPS ENSURE THAT THE SKILLS BEING DEVELOPED WILL TRANSFER TO ACADEMIC PERFORMANCE.

Students in my handwriting workshop are asked to pick one assignment during which they will practice their new handwriting skill each day. If they are getting graded on handwriting at school, that would be a good time to practice the new skills. Choose an assignment that will take about ten minutes to complete.

TROUBLESHOOTING

Once in a while the proper position of the letters is not possible because the student is not developmentally ready to write in the space provided. When this happens, try using wider spaced lines or try to do the writing activity on a large chalkboard or dry erase board. If the student cannot hold the pencil, try using a fatter pencil.

If the student has extreme difficulty maintaining good posture during the procedure, there may be a problem with muscle tonicity. His primitive reflexes should be checked, along with his sensory integration ability. In these cases, your optometrist can refer you to an occupational therapist who is well-trained in the areas of sensory integration and primitive reflexes.

SUMMARY

Good handwriting can be achieved with practice. Proper posture, correct positioning of body and hand, natural breathing, materials, proper grip of pencil, and guiding movement with the eyes are required to achieve proper handwriting. Practice daily to gain automaticity; this will make the chore of handwriting effortless. This will have a positive effect on composition because the student will be freer to write longer sentences and use bigger words.

REVIEW

Visual skills specific for handwriting:

- Pursuits
- Clear focus
- Single vision
- Peripheral vision
- Hand/eye coordination

Time: 10 - 15 minutes daily

Coaching: Point out what is being done correctly. State what needs to be improved with guidance and positive words.

Components

- Body Position
- Proper Paper
- Pencil and Grip
- Breathing
- Soft Touch
- Eyes Lead the Hand
- Up and Over

Building Handwriting Skills

- Paper Crunch
- Finger Lift

- Paper Tear
- Clay Finger Roll
- Baton Twirl
- Card Shuffle

Practice

- Get the fingers ready to write by doing five minutes of techniques in the "Building Handwriting Skills" section
- Learn three letters of the alphabet daily
- At the end of each session, connect the letters
- Use the new technique with one subject in the classroom

Troubleshooting: Modify components as needed.

- Fatter writing utensil
- Wider spaced lines on paper
- Dry-erase board or chalkboard

5

VISUAL SECRETS FOR SPELLING

MISSPELLED WORDS CAN GIVE A NEGATIVE FIRST IMPRESSION

When our spelling is perfect, it's invisible. But when it's flawed, it prompts strong negative associations.

— Marilyn vos Savant

Spelling skills are quickly becoming lost with the advent of computer spell-check programs. Many students ask, "Why learn to spell if the computer will do it for me?" Just as with handwriting, common spelling errors lead the reader to make a judgment of the intelligence of the writer, and also of his attention to detail. Spelling is one of the first assessments of one's work that students receive upon entering school. Students quickly learn who the "good" spellers are in their class, receiving 100 percent each time, and who the poor spellers are with red marks all over their pages. Earning 100 percent on every spelling test is possible for all students. This success helps build the students' confidence in their learning ability and gives them a positive attitude toward learning. Students who practice spelling words only to fail each week's test learn that trying hard does not lead to success, but only to frustration. Ideas on how to build a student's self-confidence are discussed further in Chapter 11.

> THE BRAIN FILLS IN OR REORGANIZES THE INFORMATION TO GAIN MEANING.

Another myth about spelling is that you must be a good speller in order to be a good reader. There are many very poor spellers who love to read. In fact, good readers do not need to read all of the letters of every word to know what it says. The brain fills in or reorganizes the information to gain meaning.[29]

"Aoccdrnig to rscheearch at Cmabridge uinervtisy, it deosn't mttaer in waht oredr the ltteers in a wrod are, the olny iprmoetnt tihng is taht the frist and lsat ltteer be at the rghit pclae. The rset can be a toatl mses and you can sitll raed it wouthit porbelm. Tihs is bcuseae the huamn mnid deos not raed ervey lteter by istlef, but the wrod as a wlohe." [29]

VISUAL SKILLS FOR SPELLING

Crucial visual skills for learning to spell words correctly are as follows:

Visual Skill	Definition
Visualization	The ability to see pictures of objects with the eyes closed
Imagery	The ability to imagine in the "mind's eye" what an object looks like
Visual Memory	The ability to recall a visual picture or image viewed previously
Visual Sequential Memory	Being able to recall letters, numbers, or objects in the correct order

Non-Imagery Spatial Processing, or Aphantasia	Recalling information accurately by using a form of spatial memory that is not an image or picture
Visual Discrimination of Size, Space and Shape	The ability to see slight differences of size, space, and shape

Visualization: Students with this skill are visualizers, and can see previously-viewed items in their minds as if they were pictures.

Imagery: Students who imagine an object without being able to picture it with eyes closed will report seeing black. This is referred to as aphantasia.

Visual memory: An example of this would be the ability to see a favorite toy and describe what it looks like, as if looking at a photograph of it. There are both short-term and long-term types of visual memory skills. When a student has poor ability to visualize and no short-term visual memory, he has difficulty remembering spelling words.

Visual sequential memory: A student with difficulty in this area gets all of the letters correct but cannot recall the correct order.

Non-Imagery Spatial Processing: This is also beginning to be referred to as aphantasia.[30] The visualizers and aphantasics use very different processing techniques to recall information. Your optometrist can test your student to determine which skill is present. (Most often it is one or the other.) It is rare for a student to be able to do both types of visual processing. It is possible that individuals who develop speed-reading techniques may be aphantasics, since visualizing and subvocalization (sounding the words out in one's head) while reading is a slower process.

Visual Discrimination of Size, Space and Shape: The ability to notice differences between correctly-spelled and incorrectly-spelled words.

Good reader, poor speller.

Susie was a voracious reader and loved math, yet she had extreme difficulty with spelling. She studied her spelling words for hours, but her teacher returned her essays with red marks from the many misspelled words. Her poor spelling was bringing her grades down. Susie worked hard to learn new spelling skills by using the Visual Secrets. In just three weeks her preparation time for spelling tests decreased to 30 minutes and she was getting 100% on all of her spelling tests. She tackled her commonly misspelled words and was able to relearn how to spell them correctly. Her spelling confidence grew, and her essay writing grades improved to all A's.

UNDERSTANDING THE VISUALIZATION AND IMAGERY INFORMATION PROCESSING SYSTEMS

Optometric Vision Therapy has helped many students access the visualization information processing system and the imagery information processing system. These two systems help the student recall visual information as needed.

To help develop visualization skills in a small child, it is a good idea to tell descriptive stories without a book. Encourage small children to add to the story. When my kids were small, I would tell them a story at bedtime. They became so accustomed to the creative stories they would ask, "Mommy can you read me a story without the book?"

Another example of the visualization information processing system is as follows: Have the child close his eyes and ask him if he can see an ice cream cone. If he says yes, have him describe it. If he uses descriptive terms such as a pointed bottom or round scoops, and/or uses his hands to describe what he sees, he most likely sees the actual image.

The child who says he sees only black has difficulty describing the ice cream cone. He can only imagine it, and must use his "non-visual" memory to recall the details. This is an example of the imagery information processing system.

———⟞⟐⟐⟞———

My personal experience when communicating with individuals who process and recall visual information differently has been rather interesting. Those people who make visual pictures in their minds of what is viewed cannot comprehend what it is like to not be able to make a picture. Individuals who do not see pictures in their minds do not really believe it is possible do so. This is why consulting with an expert on the subject can reduce one's confusion.

It is easier for a coach who can visualize to teach a student who can visualize, and for an aphantasic coach to teach an aphantasic student. If this is not possible, it is important to understand which ability students use to learn spelling words. It is easier to teach students younger than 12 years old to make a visual picture of spelling words. If needed, non-imagery spatial processing can efficiently take the place of visual imagery.

When my mom was 65 years old, she took a course by Tony Robbins to learn to make visual pictures. She was always a top student and loved to read. Being an optometrist, she wanted to better understand the entire idea of visual imagery. In Robbins' course, she even walked on hot coals to help understand how to make a visual picture, but she never was able to actually see an image. Two of my very intelligent, well-read, dynamic mentors also claimed to be unable to make visual images. After many discussions about this fascinating subject, I can comfortably explain to my aphantasic students that it is okay to process and recall the presented visual information spatially instead of visually. Spatial recall can be more efficient and more rapid than visual recall.

TIME NEEDED

Once the coach and the student become familiar with the Visual Secrets for Spelling described below, it will take fifteen minutes or less to learn 10 spelling words. Spend five to ten minutes doing the techniques to get the eye-brain process ready to spell. Use proper posture and learning environment as discussed in Chapter 2.

COACHING

Students will try harder to figure out the correct letter sequence when they are curious to know. Telling them they got the word wrong is defeating. It is critical to define what is correct about the attempt to spell the word, not that the whole word is wrong. The coaching method can be learned from reading a book written in 1974 called *Liberated Parents, Liberated Children: Your Guide to a Happier Family* by Adele Faber and Elaine Mazlish. This book helps you as a coach to state when the correct answer is given, and when to ask probing questions so the student can discover the correct answer.

> TELLING A STUDENT HE GOT THE WORD WRONG IS DEFEATING. IT IS CRITICAL TO DEFINE WHAT IS CORRECT ABOUT THE ATTEMPT TO SPELL THE WORD, NOT THAT THE WHOLE WORD IS WRONG.

COMPONENTS OF SPELLING

Syllables

Did you know that there is a vowel in almost every syllable in the English language? It is true. There is one word, however, that has two syllables and only one vowel. Do you know what the word is? Look at the end of this section for the answer.

Vowels

Parents and coaches, it's important for your student to know how to determine the number of syllables in the word he's learning to spell. Also be sure the student knows what vowels are: *A, E, I, O, U* and sometimes *Y*. When spelling a word, the number of vowels will be equal to or greater than the number of syllables. Many students do not know this, so have a discussion about it and give them some examples to figure out. Use the student's name or use a word like Mississippi to illustrate this concept. Also point out there can be more vowels than syllables, but not more syllables than vowels. After writing or verbally spelling a word, the student should check to ensure there is at least one vowel in each syllable.

THE MONTECALVO SPELLING TECHNIQUE

The word the student will learn is, Montecalvo (pronounced Mon-tee-kal-voe). Yes, that is my last name. I was fortunate to marry a wonderful man with a last name perfectly suited for this exercise. That is why I now refer to this spelling technique as The MONTECALVO Spelling Technique.

Materials:

- Coach's two hands
- Paper and pencil

Procedure:

Step 1: Count the syllables in Montecalvo. Have your student say each syllable separately, overemphasizing the sounds of the letters in each syllable. It sounds like, MON-TE-CAL-VO. The answer is four syllables.

Step 2: Ask, "What is the first syllable, and how many letters do you think are in that syllable?" The syllable is *Mon*, and the answer is three letters. Now, if by chance the student gives a different answer than three, do not say, "You're wrong," or "No, there are three." Instead, say, "You are close." The reason for this is to create a positive curiosity of how to find the right answer. So, if the answer he gives for *Mon* is wrong, then help the student figure it out by saying very slowly the three sounds. "M . . . o . . . n." After the student determines that he is hearing three sounds and can relate them to each letter, have the student list the three letters that represent the three sounds. If one letter is incorrect, say, "You have two of the three letters correct." Then over emphasize the sound of the one missed to see if he can identify it.

Step 3: Once the student correctly identifies the letters of the first syllable, hold up three fingers (pinky, ring, and middle) of your right hand. The coach is to state that the pinky represents *M*, ring finger represents *O* and the middle finger represents *N*. Now wiggle pinky and ask, "Which letter is this?" The student should respond, "M." Then wiggle your ring finger and have the student label that finger *O*. The middle finger is then labeled *N*. Repeat in a different order: wiggle ring finger, the student reports *O*; wiggle middle finger, student reports *N*; then wiggle your pinky and the response is *M*.

Step 4: The second syllable. It is done the same way as *Mon* but with *te* instead. *T* is represented by the right pointer and *E* is represented by the right thumb. Randomly wiggle each finger of the right hand and have your student correctly identify the letter associated with that finger. Often with *te*, the student says there is only one letter. Remind him of the rule that there is always a vowel in each syllable. They may guess which vowel fits. Overemphasize the *E* sound so they can correctly identify the vowel. If the student guesses *I*, say that would sound like *tie*; use sounds like *too*, *ta*, etc., to help your student hear the correct sound and relate it to *te*.

Step 5: The third syllable is *cal*. These letters are associated as follows: *C* is represented by your left thumb, *A* by your left pointer, and *L* by your left middle finger. After *Mon*, *te*, and *cal* are associated with the correct fingers, randomly wiggle each one so the student can quickly and correctly call out the letter associated with it. If there is a miss-call, then go back and forth between the missed letter and the letter immediately following it until they are both always correctly identified quickly and easily. This creates an automatic visual recall that solidifies the correct sequence. The term for this recall is *automaticity*.

Step 6: The fourth syllable is *vo*. These letters are associated as follows: *V* is the left ring finger and *O* is the left pinky. Once all ten letters have correct representations, randomly wiggle them so all can be easily identified without error.

Step 7: When fairly confident that the student can easily identify the random sequence of the letters, have the student spell *Montecalvo* in order, from *M* to the final *O*, while wiggling the correct finger associated with each letter. Then spell the word backward from *O* to *M*, wiggling the correct finger as the student spells backward. Let the student self-correct by stopping and re-wiggling the finger that is miss-called. Remember, *never* say "No" or "You're wrong." Once the student can accomplish this without error, ask him to very quickly spell the word forward and backward without hesitation. This again creates automaticity, which improves long-term memory for the spelled word.

Step 8: After spelling forward and backward is easy and effortless, remove the fingers and have the student spell the word without looking at the wiggling fingers. State that there are ten letters in *Montecalvo*. Ask the student, "Which one is the first letter?" He should answer with ease, "M." Then ask, "Which is the tenth letter? The third? The seventh?", etc. Ask randomly all numbers until it is easy to answer the correct letter by its numerical order.

Practice the student's weekly spelling list during the weekend before the test will be given. Most teachers give a practice test on Wednesday and the final one on Friday. Some teachers allow students to skip the Friday test if all the words are correct on Wednesday. When this is the case, our goal for the students is to get 100% on Wednesday so that he does not need to take the test on Friday. This is a big win and a huge confidence builder for the student. The whole class knows who gets free time while the others have to take the test.

If your student does not receive the words until Monday of the same week the test is given, ask to receive it on the preceding Friday. This gives you time to work on the words over the weekend. Most teachers will comply. This can also be written into an Individualized Education Plan (IEP). A good idea is to have a copy of the spelling list in the car. Tape it to the dashboard so it doesn't get lost to help you review the words. Then, when you are driving to an activity, the list will be handy and your student can practice the words in the car. Every Sunday we practiced our three kids' spelling lists on the way to church. This saved time for the whole family.

BUILDING SPELLING SKILLS

To help students become better spellers, work on their sequencing abilities early on. Here are some activities that can help develop visual sequence and visual discrimination skills.

1. Stacking Cups

Materials:

- Stacking Cup Set

Procedure:

Step 1: Place the cups randomly on the table or floor, with the largest one in the center nearest to the student, who should be seated comfortably.

Step 2: Ask the student to find the next-largest cup and put it into the biggest one. Repeat with the next-largest one, and so on until all the cups are fitted inside of each other.

Step 3: Repeat Step 1, except have all cups upside down.

Step 4: To build a tower, put the second-largest cup on top of the biggest one. Repeat with the next largest one, and so on until all are stacked, making a tower.

2. Parquetry Block Memory

Materials:

- Parquetry Block Set
- 8" x 11" card made of poster board

Procedure:

Step 1. Make two equal sets of blocks, one for the coach and one for the student.

Step 2. Make a design using two blocks. Position the 8" x 11" card so the student cannot see the design being made. The blocks are placed in a horizontal row.

Step 3. Show the design for five seconds, then cover it with the card.

Step 4. Have the student make the design to match the one under the card.

Step 5. Repeat with the same number of blocks until it is easy. Then add another block and repeat Steps 1 through 4. Increase the number of blocks up to 8.

First, make your designs easy to remember. An example would be a house with one square and one triangle for the roof. After the activity becomes easy, place your blocks in a row. Sometimes have them touch, and sometimes have them separated by either an equal amount of space between the blocks, or a varied amount. Be sure the design made by the student matches exactly.

PRACTICING

SPELLING TEST

Now it is time to give a practice spelling test at home. It is important to learn how the student's teacher gives the test in school. How do they say the word? Is it given in a sentence?

Materials:

- Paper

- Pencil

Procedure

Step 1: Give the test the exact same way the student's teacher gives it. After the test is completed, the student gets to correct his work.

Step 2: Have the student tell the coach how the word was spelled by calling out each letter. If the word is correct, have the student draw a star by the word. If the word is missing a letter or they are in the incorrect sequence, tell the student what part of the word is correct. An example would be "You got six of the seven letters right," or, "You got all of the seven letters right, and five are in the right place." Then have the student circle the word so it can be re-learned with The MONTECALVO Spelling Technique.

Step 3: After checking the spelling, have the student re-learn the ones circled, then retake the entire test, including the words with stars. After all of the words can be spelled correctly in one sitting, do not worry about practicing the words until the night before the test. Most often, the words will be retained.

Step 4: Retake the same spelling test the night before the classroom test. Relearn any words that are not correct.

—◦◦◦—

The exciting thing about using The MONTECALVO Spelling Technique with students who are in third grade or below is that, after about a year, they will be able to read their spelling words and immediately know how to spell them forward and backward without practice. They may need to work on one or two from time to time, but for the most part, learning their weekly words may take less than ten minutes. Students in fifth grade or older will be able to learn their words automatically after using this technique for two to four months. By the time they are in middle school with a long list of difficult words, they will have the skills to learn the words quickly while other students who don't know the Visual Secrets for Spelling will need more time to learn them. Your student will then be able to dedicate more time to learning other more complicated subjects such as algebra, literature, and history.

> CHILDREN IN FIFTH GRADE OR OLDER WILL BE ABLE TO LEARN THEIR WORDS AUTOMATICALLY AFTER USING THIS TECHNIQUE FOR TWO TO FOUR MONTHS.

Parent coaches should try this technique. It is enjoyable to challenge the adults in my workshops to do five words a day for two weeks. With the brain's unique neuroplasticity, adults will be able to easily spell words forward and backward with little effort in a short amount of time.

TROUBLESHOOTING

Besides weekly spelling tests, students commonly misspell words in writing assignments. It is important to stop repeatedly misspelling the same word, which teaches the brain to spell the word incorrectly each time it is written. Every time the eyes send the incorrect sequence of letters to the brain, that improper sequence is reinforced. Undoing this is much more work than learning to spell it correctly in the first place. Students with high IQs and poor spelling habits may have a much harder time un-learning misspelled words because they can have greater difficulty letting go of poor habits.

I ride my horse in an outdoor corral, but she often wants to leave the corral and return to the barn. If I let her turn toward the exit gate (because she wants to stop working), it takes me 15 rounds of preventing her from turning toward the gate to stop the habit. This is similar to teaching a student to relearn a misspelled word.

To change these habits, the following technique will help resolve the commonly misspelled words. This technique allows for the eye-brain process to only see the correctly sequenced word. The student should not write or see the incorrect sequence.

COMMONLY MISSPELLED WORDS

Materials:

- 3" x 5" index card
- Medium tip black marker

Procedure:

Step 1: Make a list of the commonly misspelled words.

Step 2: Choose 5 to 10 words to work on each week. The number you choose depends on age and how much other homework the student is asked to complete at home. Summertime may be a good time to fix these misspelled words.

Step 3: Use The MONTECALVO Spelling Technique to learn and practice the correct sequence of the letters in each word.

Step 4: Write the list of 5 to 10 words on a 3" x 5" index card in lower case letters with the marker.

Step 5: Explain to the teacher the student will use the card of commonly-misspelled words when he chooses to write one of the words in any of his subjects. He will copy the word instead of writing it from memory, which will reinforce the correct spelling in his brain.

Step 6: Repeat each week with a new set of words from the list of commonly misspelled words.

SUMMARY

Your student can learn to improve spelling skills. Break words into syllables, and learn the sequence of the letters of each syllable. Repeat the letters both randomly and in order until there are no errors. Write the word correctly every time to avoid seeing the incorrect sequence. Spelling can be improved at any age. The MONTECALVO Spelling Technique has helped students improve their spelling skills. It can help your student too.

Were you able to come up with the answer to the question, "What word has two syllables but one vowel?" The answer is *rhythm*.

REVIEW

Visual Skills

- Visualization

- Visual Memory

- Visual Sequential Memory
- Non-Imagery Spatial Processing

TIME NEEDED

Fifteen minutes per week to learn ten words. Fifteen minutes to take and correct the practice spelling test. Once The MONTECALVO Spelling Technique becomes automatic, learning the spelling words and taking the practice test may go quicker.

COACHING

State which letters are correct in the attempted spelling word. Explain if a few are out of sequence. State how many letters are missing.

Components

- Vowels
- Syllables
- The MONTECALVO Spelling Technique

Building Spelling Skills

- Stacking Cups
- Parquetry Block Memory

Practice

- Use The MONTECALVO Spelling Technique to learn how to spell words
- Practice test

- Re-learn words if needed

- Re-take test

- Do one more practice test the night before an in-class test

Troubleshooting

- List commonly misspelled words

- Pick 5 to 10 to learn in one week

- Use The MONTECALVO Spelling Technique to learn words

- Take a practice test

- Write on a 3" x 5" index card for regular reference

6

VISUAL SECRETS FOR COMPOSITION

GREAT WRITERS WIN SCHOLARSHIPS

Good writing is clear, concise and correct. Great writing captivates, engages and motivates.

— Lisa Horn

Why should one want to be a good writer? The answer is because writing is an important skill for accurate communication of thoughts and ideas. The written word lasts much longer than the spoken word and allows for those who have read it to go back and review it easily. Your important ideas will not be lost after they are written down.

When my three kids were young they were fairly good at grammar, but writing creative stories proved more difficult for them. All of them excelled at science and math, which may be the reason why they aren't as naturally skilled in creative writing. To help my kids, I enlisted the help of a college student who was working on a creative writing degree. She would come to our home and take my kids down to the stream in the woods to write. She gave them special notebooks and pens to use. There, she asked them to write about anything they wanted. There were prompts, but no grammar corrections and no emphasis on spelling. In a few short weeks, they began to develop better creative writing skills. I saved the stories and still enjoy reading them today.

Problems with composition are evident when a student:

- writes short sentences absent of adjectives or adverbs

- verbally cannot use full sentences with ease

- cannot make up an imaginary story and tell it verbally

- cannot verbally describe familiar objects

The ability to communicate one's thoughts into written form is a skill that is often stifled when spelling, handwriting, and grammar are emphasized at the same time. If a student has difficulty with any of these skills, he will learn that easy words and short sentences can get the job done with fewer red ink marks from the teacher. This shortcut solution suppresses creativity at an early age, and it becomes difficult to revive later on.

THE ABILITY TO COMMUNICATE ONE'S THOUGHTS INTO WRITTEN FORM IS A SKILL THAT IS OFTEN STIFLED WHEN SPELLING, HANDWRITING, AND GRAMMAR ARE EMPHASIZED AT THE SAME TIME.

Another issue that can interfere with composition is minimal use of oral language. When students use hand gestures or head nods, or wait for someone else to answer for them, they are not learning to develop important verbal and vocabulary skills. Well-developed verbal skills help students organize their thoughts so they can transfer their ideas to paper with ease. Using verbal language frequently also allows for vocabulary building and better verbal expression.

Not only will this help build writing skills, it also has an added benefit when it comes time to interview for a job or a post-graduate position. It is important to encourage even young children to use full sentences with many adjectives and adverbs to describe what they are speaking about. Verbal skills can improve by participating in a few easy activities and can be transferred to quality composition.

This chapter on composition discusses how to improve a student's ability to compose interesting, creative responses and more accurate technical answers when needed. Two main categories of writing are creative and technical. The good news is, there is a place in this world for both. If one needs to write a story for scholarships or for a college application, having creative writing skills is a huge advantage. When applying for a job, writing grants or proofreading scientific or instructional documents, technical writing skills are more helpful.

English, history and language arts are subjects where creative writing is most often used for describing one's ideas. Science and math are subjects in which technical writing is preferred for communicating one's thoughts.

VISUAL SKILLS FOR COMPOSITION

Visual skills specific to composition are as follows:

Visual Skill	Definition
Visualization or Visual Imagery	The ability to see or imagine with the mind's eye
Visual Memory	Being able to recall previously viewed information or scenes
Visual Closure	The ability to finish an idea or to complete a partially drawn picture
Visual Identification, Matching and Discrimination of Size, Shape, and Space	Knowing similarities and differences of what is being thought of or looked at
Visual Association	Relating one idea to another

Visual Categorization	Grouping similar items or ideas together

Visualization: The ability to picture either an image or a scene guides a writer to put those ideas, thoughts, and images into words.

Visual Memory: Important for when you want to remember the details about what has been read or experienced. This skill is also helpful for completing an essay about recently-learned material.

Visual Closure: If you see a scene, Visual Closure allows you to anticipate what might be next. This is helpful in creative writing.

Visual Identification, Matching, and Discrimination of Size, Shape, and Space: The ability to notice what goes together and what does not. This is beneficial when organizing the content being written.

Visual Association: An example is when you flip a light switch and the light turns on. You relate the switch to the light.

Visual Categorization: Helps the student group ideas. This is useful when composing a paragraph so the student's writing flows well.

Mary couldn't write well.

Mary learned at an early age that if she wrote short sentences with small words, her assignments wouldn't come back with lots of red marks that corrected her grammatical errors. Now in middle school her new English teacher wanted creative essays. She was struggling to figure out what to write about and how to write it. Mary followed the Visual Secrets for composition, and after a few months she was able to compose more interesting essays. She even entered a writing contest.

TIME NEEDED

Once the student is comfortable with composing, spend about 30 minutes practicing creative writing skills. If the student gets caught up in composing and goes longer, that will be a huge win.

COACHING

Do not correct grammar or spelling while practicing composition. Build creativity daily by asking lots of questions and waiting as long as needed to get a complete verbal response.

PRACTICE

The student will be developing new positive writing experiences. He will be doing a little more each session. This will ease him into being more comfortable with regular creative writing assignments.

COMPOSING

Materials:

- Quiet designated writing time
- Dictionary
- Thesaurus
- Fun writing utensil
- Quality paper
- Computer
- Comfortable creative environment
  - Desk
  - Chair
  - Lighting

Procedure:

Step 1: Have the student write one sentence every day for one week.

Step 2: Then write one paragraph every day for the second week. The sentences and paragraphs do not need to relate to one another.

Step 3: In the third week, write one sentence every day about something about which you know nothing. Make up ideas, items, or concepts.

Step 4: The fourth week, write a paragraph regarding something about which you know nothing. Make up ideas, items, or concepts.

Step 5: For week five, write a one-page story about something personally important to you. Try to be very descriptive.

Step 6: During week six, go back and re-write the sentences from week one, making them more interesting by adding descriptive words to the nouns and verbs.

Step 7: For week seven, rewrite the sentences from week six and make them sound scary.

Step 8: For week eight, rewrite the sentences from week six and make them sound funny.

These activities will teach the student how to manipulate the written word, and create different impressions by using better descriptive words. Grammar, spelling or handwriting errors should *not* be corrected for these activities. If your student does not know how to spell a word, simply tell him how to spell it (instead of making him look it up, which can stifle the creative thought). Let the student use a thesaurus to look up adjectives and adverbs. Encourage the student to use different words that mean the same thing.

LET THE STUDENT USE A THESAURUS TO LOOK UP ADJECTIVES AND ADVERBS. ENCOURAGE THE STUDENT TO USE DIFFERENT WORDS THAT MEAN THE SAME THING.

BUILDING COMPOSITION SKILLS

1. Visual/Verbal Description

This activity is accomplished by having the student describe something in the room. The coach tries to determine what is being described. Be sure to wait until lots of good descriptive words are being used so there is no question of what and where the item is. Encourage words that describe size, shape, color, and location.

2. Story Telling

Choose a word around which to create a story. For example, ask the student to tell a story about the word *basket*. He gets one point for every sentence that has five words, and one additional point each time he includes the word *basket*. He gets five points when he uses a ten-word sentence.

3. Using Full Sentences

Designate a specific time frame, such as 30 minutes, during which all conversation must be full sentences of more than three words. When the student uses a sentence or phrase of less than three words, the student loses a point. If he uses a sentence of greater than three words, he gains a point. As the student gets better at this activity, designate longer and longer times you ask him to use full sentences.

4. Describing an Object

Ask the student to describe an object in such a way that an alien from another planet would know exactly what it was. Example: The object is an apple. Say, "Describe an apple but do not use the word fruit." The student may say, "The item is red." The coach responds, "Is it a fire truck?" This will usually gain a little laughter. The goal is to ask questions so the student can

85

discover how to better describe the object. The questions are used to guide the student and make the experience positive. As the student gains confidence in this activity, have him begin responding in full sentences. Encourage the student to use as many descriptive words as possible for each sentence. These words might be specific about color, size, or weight. They might be words like *inside, outside, bright,* or *dull.*

5. Describing an Activity

Ask the student to describe an activity in extreme detail so a stranger could complete it perfectly without help. For example, "How do I set the table at your house?" The student may say, "I put the plates on the table." Your response should be, "Which plates? What color? Where are they? How many?" The goal is for the coach to ask very few questions, because your student's description will permit you to know exactly how to carry out the task.

6. Thesaurus Word Game

Pick an adjective like *good.* Ask the student how many words he can think of that mean *good.* Use common words like nice, beautiful, helpful, etc. to build his vocabulary. Do the same with adverbs such as *slowly, quickly,* etc.

TROUBLESHOOTING

Some students may have extreme difficulty using words verbally and then transferring them to a composition task. They have either not developed creative thinking, or it has been stifled by stress. Shy children and introverts have more difficulty with learning to use words verbally. To help this type of challenge, decrease the complexity of the ideas discussed above by requiring fewer words. Pick up some board games that require speaking. Clue is an example of a game where the player needs to ask other players questions to determine the final answer. Other games are I Spy, Scattergories, and Fact or Fiction.

SUMMARY

There are many ways to improve a student's ability to compose. The key is to be supportive of his or her efforts and to remove the pressure by not requiring perfect grammar, spelling, or sentence structure. Use lots of language communication to develop the student's thinking ability so he can eventually put those ideas into the written word. Once the student gains confidence, many roadblocks will be removed.

REVIEW

Visual Skills for Composition

- Visualization or Visual Imagery
- Visual Memory
- Visual Closure
- Visual Identification, Matching, and Discrimination of Size, Shape and Space
- Visual Association
- Visual Categorization

Time Needed

- 30 minutes daily

Coaching

- Ask questions
- Don't correct grammar or spelling

Practice

- Write one sentence per week
- Write one paragraph per week
- Write sentences about an unknown subject
- Write paragraphs about an unknown subject
- Write a one-page personal story
- Add adjectives and adverbs to sentences for more interest
- Rewrite interesting sentences, making them scary
- Rewrite interesting sentences, making them funny

Building Skills

- Visual/Verbal Description
- Story Telling
- Using Full Sentences
- Describing Objects
- Describing an Activity

Troubleshooting:

Play games to reduce stress and increase speaking ability

- Clue
- I Spy
- Scattergories
- Fact or Fiction

7

VISUAL SECRETS FOR MATH

BETTER JOB WITH EXCEPTIONAL MATHEMATICS SKILLS

*To understand the universe you must know
the language in which it is written—and
that language is mathematics.*

— Galileo Galilei

Many professions, from entry-level to high-level positions, require simple mathematical skills. Carpenters use math all the time to decide how long a board needs to be. They need to know where to make cuts to create the least amount of waste. Builders calculate the area of a room for such things as ceiling tiles and carpet. Retail checkout employees need to be able to understand percentages to figure out how much to discount the original price when there is a sale. Engineers, accountants, optometrists, and pharmacists are a few of many professions that require higher-level math skills. Being good at math allows the student to have a full array of opportunities when choosing a future career.

The goal of math is to solve problems; however, when we look at the problems that are being solved, we must understand that math is about measuring space in many different ways. Numbers are used to represent different amounts of space. To make this easy for learning the basics, we will only be using linear examples of math. This means that the amount of *space* represented by each number is the same and the distance between (or the *space* between) numbers is always equal.

Learning math facts, such as multiplication tables, is simply a memorization activity and is not really math. Automaticity is used for this memorization skill. Using numbers does not always equal the building of math concepts. To build math concepts one must understand what numbers represent and then learn how to manipulate them to measure or calculate the space they occupy.

Note that, indeed, math facts are important. They help students complete math homework in a shorter amount of time. During math tests the student can focus on the actual problem instead of taking longer to figure out a math fact. Knowing math facts also helps to do math problems in your head.

Automaticity is the ability to complete a task with minimal effort and little thought. For example, when driving to work the same way every day, you may go into an automatic mode. You stop at the traffic lights when they are red, and go when they are green. When you get to work, you may remember little about the drive if it was uneventful. You drove safely in an automatic mode. Another example is when you are very good at a sport and are playing and making goals without thinking and little effort. You are playing "in the zone," and you are using automaticity. When you first learn to drive a car with a manual transmission, each action requires thought and takes effort. After getting good at driving a car with a stick shift, you do not have to think about each individual step. Similarly, automaticity allows for the child to memorize math facts without effort.

IF KNOWING MATH FACTS IS SIMPLY MEMORIZATION AND ISN'T REALLY MATH, WHY IS IT IMPORTANT?

Memorization of math facts helps save time when taking higher-level math classes such as algebra, geometry, and calculus. Knowing the answers to math facts makes valuable homework time shorter. Doing math in one's head quickly is a good skill to develop at an early age. By the time my son got to high school, he was quite good at doing math in his head. One day his sister asked to borrow his calculator for algebra. He replied, "I don't have one." Hearing this, I asked him, "You are taking tenth-grade geometry! How do you do your homework without a calculator?" His response was that he just did the calculations in his head.

> MEMORIZATION OF MATH FACTS HELPS SAVE TIME WHEN TAKING HIGHER-LEVEL MATH CLASSES SUCH AS ALGEBRA, GEOMETRY, AND CALCULUS.

VISUAL SKILLS FOR MATH

Visual skills specific to math are described in this table:

Visual Skill	Definition
Binocularity	The ability to use our two eyes together so they send the same message to the brain at the same time
Laterality and Directionality	Knowing one's sidedness (right or left, top or bottom, front or back); Positioning and relating to the world around you
Spatial Organization and Orientation	The ability to arrange information and relate it to one's self and surroundings
Visual Closure	Being able to fill in missing information to understand what is being viewed

Visual Figure Ground	Being aware of an object viewed without letting the background interfere
Association	The ability to see how one object relates to another
Categorization	Being able to put similar objects together

Binocularity: Depth perception, or 3D viewing, is completely dependent on binocularity. Binocularity relates to higher math when perceiving and rotating objects in order to measure them. Those who do not have depth perception have difficulty with these tasks. Compared to 40 years ago, hundreds more jobs today are dependent upon depth perception, especially in the field of engineering.

Laterality and Directionality: The concepts of right and left and the cardinal directions (North, South, East, West) are dependent upon this visual skill. Knowing these concepts is critical to understanding visual space. Since math entails measuring space in many different ways, the student needs a foundation, which is "self," from which to reference visual space.

Spatial Organization and Orientation: The abilities to arrange information and relate it to self and surroundings. These abilities will serve the student well when trying to figure out geometry and calculus.

Visual Closure: This helps in solving math problems and story problems.

Figure Ground: Differentiating figure (center) from ground (peripheral) is critical for math to determine what part of the problem is important to pay attention to and what is less important.

Association: Important when grouping things that have something in common.

Categorization: When doing sets and subsets this skill is helpful. This helps build a foundation for more complex mathematical structures.

Steven hated math.

He especially disliked the timed tests. Each night his parents struggled to help him finish his math homework. He just did not remember the concepts. After taking Steven for a comprehensive optometric evaluation with a doctor that specialized in vision therapy, it was determined that he had difficulty with spatial concepts and laterality. After developing these skills, he then completed the activities for math in *Visual Secrets for School Success*. He began to understand what numbers meant. He learned an easy way to remember math facts and he began getting better grades on his timed tests. Although he had some catching up to do, he was eventually able to understand math concepts such as fractions and decimals. Several years later he earned an "A" in geometry class.

TIME

Working on math concepts should take only 20 minutes per day. More time than that can be overwhelming for students. In addition to spending time on math concept-building, incorporate games and counting equal-sized objects into daily activities when possible.

COACHING

If the answer you receive is not the correct one, you need to figure out how to ask questions so the student can discover the right answer. Continued repetition builds memorization and does not help him understand the concept. If there are many errors at the level being worked on, reduce the level of complexity.

When correcting math papers, tell the student how many problems are *correct*. If all are correct, the student is finished with the assignment. When there are incorrect answers, have the student figure out which ones are incorrect. You do not tell the student which ones are right or wrong... he should tell *you*. Give a big reward when he gets 100 percent correct.

We used a "treasure chest" reward system for our kids. If they were able to achieve 100% on an assignment, they got to pick a prize. This worked great for Andrew, who began to take more time checking his work to ensure all answers were correct before he handed it in. The teacher commented on how hard he worked to be sure that every answer was correct.

COMPONENTS AND CONCEPTS

- Linear Units

- Multiplication and Division

- Fractions

LINEAR UNITS

Think about the number 1. It represents one unit of something that occupies a certain amount of space. The number 2 represents twice as much space occupied as the number 1. So, a good visual is to imagine or visualize a set of 10 equal-sized stair steps that represents each number, 1 through 10. See Illustration #7. This will create a good visual for the first activity. You can quickly check if your student has difficulty with this linear concept by asking one question: "Is the space between 2 and 3 smaller than, larger than, or equal to the space between numbers 52 and 53?" Some students think that 52 and 53 are further apart from each other than 2 and 3 are, because 52 and 53 are larger numbers. They do not understand that in linear math, the space between each consecutive number is the same.

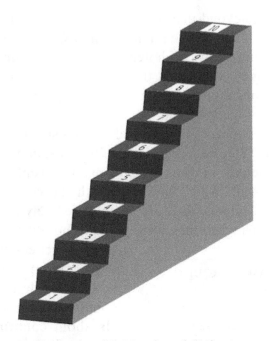

Illustration #7: Numbered Stairsteps

When the linear math concept is not developed, a student must rely on memorization to determine mathematical answers. The student does not know why or how he achieved the correct answer. Students with good memory can pass all of their math facts, giving everyone a false sense of security that they are good at math. When they get to higher math, they begin to struggle because they do not understand the basic concepts. Those who are not good at memorization learn to "hate" math because they are always pushed to memorize and are timed to prove they know their math facts. This scenario creates stress for these students.

How does one begin to develop "unit" mathematical concepts? This begins at a very young age. Remember when your student was learning to count? He would assign number 1 to the thumb of the left hand, then 2 to the pointer finger of the left hand, then count audibly from three to ten as he touched the next three fingers of the left hand. This shows he understood

1 and 2, but beyond that, the numbers 3 through 10 had no meaning. In his mind the numbers simply follow each other. When the child knows each item represents a number then he is beginning to understand the concept of numbers. This is indicated when counts accurately 1 through 5 as he touches each finger of the left hand.

The unit concept is reinforced when a small child counts his footsteps. Step counting is one of the most important activities to participate in when learning math concepts. If you ask a group of adults which ones love math and which ones hate math, those who love math are much more likely to remember counting steps when they were young. Those who hate math usually never counted steps.

> IF YOU ASK A GROUP OF ADULTS WHICH ONES LOVE MATH AND WHICH ONES HATE MATH, THOSE WHO LOVE MATH ARE MUCH MORE LIKELY TO REMEMBER COUNTING STEPS WHEN THEY WERE YOUNG.

Do you know any engineers or people really good at math? Ask these individuals about counting steps. They usually have continued to count steps into adulthood, and some never stop. Clinically, I have noticed the longer a person counts steps, the better he is at math and at being successful when using math concepts on a daily basis.

When the unit concept is not well-developed in students, they should begin counting steps everywhere they go. Counting stair steps is better at emphasizing the unit concept than counting footsteps because one can feel the same equal exertion required to lift one's body when moving from step 1 to 2 as it is when moving from step 8 to 9. The effort between numbers is equal because the steps rise equal amounts. (See the Counting Steps Activity in this chapter to develop this skill.)

I discovered the correlation between counting steps and enjoyment of math when presenting my math workshops for parents. We live near Wright-Patterson Air Force Base in Ohio, and there are many parents in my audiences who are engineers.

When asked who still counts steps as an adult, the engineers always raised their hands. Audience members who claimed to be poor at math and really disliked it didn't raise their hands.

One cold morning when the temperature was below zero, I asked my husband (who has an engineering degree), if it was too cold to walk across the street from his office to the bank during his lunch hour. His response was, "No, it is only 47 steps from door to door." Engineers, it seems, count everything.

Another way to check a student's unit concept development is to create the following situation. Place five paperclips on the table in front of your student. Ask, "How many paperclips are on the table?" If the student must count the paperclips to know how many exist, he has not developed the understanding of the unit concept. Repeat with four paperclips, then three, then two, then one, to determine which amount he can accurately identify without having to count them. To develop this, the following activities are recommended: Counting Steps, and Dice Game. See explanations of these activities below.

It is extremely important to teach the student *not* to count on his fingers to determine the answers. Why is this? On a hand, five fingers do not represent equal units. The pointer finger does not occupy two times as much space as the thumb does. The middle finger is not three times larger than the thumb. The ring finger is not four times larger than the thumb and, for sure, the pinky is not five times larger than the thumb. The other problem with learning to add and subtract with one's fingers is that it is a very hard habit to break. In subtraction you take away numbers, but you cannot take away the fingers.

Once using fingers to count becomes a habit, the student always has the temptation to use them to ensure he has the correct answer. This actually happened to my daughter in first grade. Her Montessori preschool had taught her long addition, subtraction, multiplication, and division using math manipulative techniques. When she attended first grade in a public school, however, her teacher taught her finger counting and touch point math. This technique was used to help every student achieve the right answer. My very bright daughter, unfortunately, caught on to finger counting quite quickly. Even now, though she has advanced mathematical skills, she still falls back to finger counting on occasion. Bright children have a more difficult time giving up habits that interfere with developing automatic skills.

ADDITION AND SUBTRACTION

Another way to assess understanding of the unit concept is to ask the student, "If I am standing on step 8, how many steps does it take to get to step 10?" If the student needs to count to figure it out and gives the correct answer of "Two," ask "How many from step 28 to 30?" Wait for his answer of, "Two." He might be counting it in his head. Continue to re-ask, using 38 to 40, 58 to 60, etc. Once he begins answering "Two" automatically, without hesitation, say, "Isn't it interesting that every time you are on a step that ends with an 8, there are always 2 steps to reach the step that ends in 0. What if you are on step 7—how many would it be to step 10?" What about 37 to 40, 57 to 60, etc.? Do you think there are always 3 steps between the steps ending in 7 and 0?" If the student responds *yes* and understands this idea, explain that each time you reach 0, you will start over with the same set of ten numbers, and they are the same distance apart regardless of whether they are in the 50s, 60s, 70s, or 100s. See Illustration #7. Once the concepts of the numbered stairsteps are in place, this is a good time to introduce the 100 Square Game. (See the 100 Square Game activity, this chapter.)

Once a student has successfully developed the linear concepts of numbers, we move on to understanding other math concepts which will include multiplication, division, fractions, and simple geometry. The goal is for the student to develop a visual construct of what these concepts mean in terms of how they represent space.

MULTIPLICATION AND DIVISION

With multiplication and division concepts, it is best to show a representation of "sets." Four times three means adding four sets of three equally sized items. See Illustration #8. In this illustration, you see four sets of three blocks stacked on top of each other. Ask the student how many are on the first row. Show how this represents 1 times 3, which equals 3. Then ask, "How many are in the first and second row?" Show how this represents 2 times 3, which equals 6. Continue adding sets of 3 blocks until the student understands that he needs to add 3 to each total to get the answer.

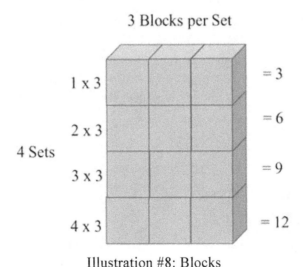

3 Blocks per Set

1 x 3 = 3

2 x 3 = 6

4 Sets

3 x 3 = 9

4 x 3 = 12

Illustration #8: Blocks

Many students dislike division, but division is the same as multiplication, only backward. To describe division, take the same illustration and show how to use different words to describe division. If there are 12 blocks, how many sets of 3 are there? How many sets of 4? When students see that multiplication and division are treated in a similar fashion, it makes both easier to accomplish.

FRACTIONS

Fractions can be confusing. To determine if the student understands fractions ask, "What is larger, 1/3 or 1/2?" If his answer is 1/3, he knows 3 is larger than 2, but is judging the size of the fraction based on the number in the denominator of the fraction. His incorrect response alerts you to the fact that a visual representation of fractions has not occurred in his mind. Present the following example to the student. You are having a pizza party on two separate nights, and you will have only one pizza for each party. You invite two friends the first night, and invite one friend the next night. At which pizza party will you get a larger piece of pizza...when you have two friends over, or one friend? Show the student by cutting some cookies in half and in thirds so he can compare the different sizes. Cookies are way more fun and tastier than felt or paper, and they improve attention for learning this concept too.

BUILDING MATH SKILLS

- Counting Steps
- Measuring Objects
- 100 Squares
- Dice Game
- Puzzles

COUNTING STEPS ACTIVITY

Materials:

- Ten stair steps that are equal in height
- Ten numbers, 1 through 10, each printed on a piece of paper

Procedure:

Step 1: Number ten steps in your house 1 through 10. See Illustration #7.

Step 2: Have the student walk forward and backward up and down the steps counting and looking at each number as he goes.

Step 3: The student stands on step number 5. Ask, "How many steps do you need to take to reach step number 8? Ask him at first to figure it out by counting the number of steps as he moves from 5 to 8. Repeat this moving forward and backward between all of the numbers.

Step 4: Once he gets good at this process ask the same question but have him figure it out in his head first, then check himself as he moves and counts between steps.

Step 5: After this is accomplished, see if he can play the next part of the game. Have him visualize or imagine the steps in his head. Have him see himself on Step 5. Call out any number 1 through 10 and he should immediately, without counting, be able to respond with the correct number of steps needed to move to the number you have called. When he can give an immediate response to any number you give him from 1 through 10, ask him to stand on step 4 and repeat. Then move to the other eight numbers and repeat.

This activity is complete when he can think of any number and know instantaneously how far that number is from the one of which he is thinking. This phase of this activity can be performed in the car when commuting to the student's various activities. This will save time and help the student complete math assignments more quickly.

MEASURING OBJECTS

Materials:

- Measuring tape
- String

Procedure:

Step 1: Give your student a measuring tape. You can either use the ones used by builders or you can get a sewing measuring tape. Cut several pieces of string of various lengths. Have your student estimate how long each string is.

Step 2: The student measures the strings with the measuring tape and discovers how closely he has estimated the string length. Repeat and see if his estimation skill improves.

Step 3: Ask how long each string will be if you cut it in half. After he gives the answer, cut the string in half and have him measure it to confirm. Repeat using 1/3, 1/4, etc.

Step 4: Ask what size the door is. Have him measure the door height and width. After learning how to calculate area with the Geoboard discussed later in this chapter, relate it to the area of the door. Measure the student's room and calculate how much carpet it would take to cover the floor.

These activities show the student how math relates to real life scenarios.

100 SQUARE GAME

Materials:

- 100 equal squares, 10 squares by 10 squares. See Illustration #9.

- 2 pennies
- 1 dime

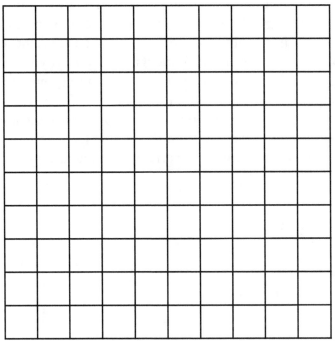

Illustration #9 – 100 Square Game

Procedure:

Step 1: The coach and the student decide what the squares represent. The first way to use the chart is to label the first upper left square with 1 or 0. If 1 is used, the top row should be labeled 1 through 10, the second row 11 through 20, the third row 21 through 30, and so on. A second way to label the chart is to make the first upper left square zero, so the top row would be numbered zero through 9, the second row would be 10 through 19, the third row 20 through 29, and so on.

Step 2: The coach and student each place a penny on the chart. The coach puts his on the top left square, and the student

103

puts his on the bottom right square. A dime is placed on a random square somewhere near the center of the chart.

Step 3: The game consists of each player taking turns moving his penny toward the dime. Play the game by moving one square each turn, and correctly calling the number of the square into which you move. You are allowed to move diagonally, horizontally, or vertically into an adjacent square. Whoever gets to the dime first gets to keep it. If your answer is incorrect, you stay where you are. If correct, remain in the new square until your next turn.

Step 4: To add complexity, have the player call out a square that is two squares away from the penny. He then moves the penny to that new square. If correct, he remains at that square until the next move.

DICE GAME

Materials

- Two large dice

Procedure:

Step 1: Throw one die on the table in front of your student, who is seated at the table.

Step 2: Ask your student to call out the number of dots he sees. Repeat by throwing the other die and have the student call out the correct number of dots that shows up. Continue until the student does not need to count the dots, but can answer with the correct response without hesitation. Once this has occurred, the student has developed automaticity in recognizing one through six.

Step 3: Repeat Steps 1 and 2, but use both dice. After this is accomplished, the student has developed automaticity of number recognition from one through 12.

PUZZLES

Students who enjoy math usually enjoy jigsaw puzzles, and those who avoid math often don't enjoy them. To build visual thinking skills important for math, encourage students to put together jigsaw puzzles. Recall my son, the engineer who loves math? When he was two years old, he could easily put together a 250-piece

STUDENTS WHO ENJOY MATH USUALLY ENJOY JIGSAW PUZZLES, AND THOSE WHO AVOID MATH OFTEN DON'T ENJOY THEM.

puzzle. He *really* liked puzzles. So, what if your student hates puzzles? The answer is to begin where he is.

Materials:

- Puzzles of varying size: 10-piece, 25-piece, 50-piece, 100-piece

- Stopwatch

Procedure:

Step 1: Find a puzzle that makes a picture of something the student likes. Begin with a 25-piece puzzle.

Step 2: Let the student try to put the puzzle together by himself. If this is too difficult, find a puzzle with fewer pieces until he can figure out how to complete it on his own. Have him repeat putting the same puzzle together multiple times. The first time a puzzle is built, it helps to build visual figure ground and visual closure. As the student becomes more familiar with the puzzle, he can put it together almost without thinking and is actually doing it from memory. He has built an important visual memory skill.

Step 3: Use a stopwatch to record the time it takes to build the puzzle the first time, and ask him to try it a second time to see if he can beat his time. Give a reward for successfully finishing the puzzle and a second reward for beating his time.

Step 4: After the 25-piece puzzle is easily accomplished quickly, try a different puzzle with the same number of pieces and repeat the above procedure until it is easy.

Step 5: When 25-piece puzzles are too easy and less fun, move to 50-piece puzzles. Once your student can quickly compete a 250-piece puzzle with little effort, he will begin to enjoy doing puzzles and continue to build these important visual skills to be used when learning math.

PRACTICING
MATH FACTS ACTIVITIES

- Body Movement and Multiplication
- Dr. M's Multiplication Technique
- Geoboard
- Parquetry Blocks
- Attribute Blocks
- Math Stars

BODY MOVEMENT AND MULTIPLICATION

Many students dislike flashcards. To help students learn math facts, coach the student to count by sets (such as 2, 4, 6, 8, 10, 12, 14, 16, 18, 20, 22, and 24) while doing a rhythmic activity such as bouncing a ball, hopping or marching. Ask the student to count by sets of two forward and backward. Next try with fives, then tens since these are easier than the other numbers. Be sure to go through all twelve sets. Once there is no hesitation with counting forward and back, try adding a metronome.

Have the student count to the beat while moving in rhythm. Once the twos are automatic, move to fives, then tens. These sets are first because they are the easiest. Next, move on to threes, fours, sixes, sevens, eights, and nines.

Dr. M's Multiplication Math Facts Technique

Step 1: The coach holds up his or her ten fingers, palms facing student. Explain to the student that each finger will represent the number of the set. The pinky finger on the right hand is set one, the ring finger is set two, the middle finger is set three, the index finger is set four, and the thumb is set five. The thumb on the left hand is set six, the index finger is set seven, the middle finger is set eight, the ring finger is set nine and the pinky finger is set ten. When the coach wiggles a finger, the student gives the answer that matches the set represented. When the coach wiggles his right pinky and you are working on sets of two, then the answer would be two: 1 x 2 = 2. If the right pointer wiggles, then the answer would be eight: 4 x 2 = 8. And so forth. First go in order: 2, 4, 6, 8, 10 and so on. Then backward: 20, 18, 16, 14, and so on. Then wiggle the fingers randomly until there is no hesitation with the answer. If one set is hard for the student to remember, go back and forth between an easy one and the one that is hard to remember until the eye-brain connection is made and the student is correct each time any finger is wiggled.

Step 2: Without using fingers, call out a number of the set you're working on and have the student give the correct answer. Example: For a set of 2, the coach says 4 and the student answers 8 without hesitation.

Step 3: Repeat Step 1 with fives and tens, then do all the other numbers. Learning multiplication with the above two activities will save your student time when it comes to solving algebraic and geometric problems in the future.

GEOBOARD

Materials

- Geoboard

- Different colored rubber bands

Procedure:

Step 1: Simple geometry can be taught by using a Geoboard. There are small ones with 25 pegs, larger ones containing 100 pegs, and each has several rubber bands. At first, do not let the student see the board. Ask him, "What is a square?" If he replies, "It has four sides," show him a rubber band surrounding 6 squares making a rectangle. Ask, "Is this a square?" He should respond *no*. You then ask, "So what is a square?" The response may be, "It has four equal sides." See Illustration # 10.

Step 2: Show the student a diamond and ask, "Is this a square?" The response should be *no*. He should then respond with, "A square has four equal sides with the same corners," or "Four equal sides with 90-degree corners." Any correct variation of the definition of a square is acceptable. Remember, do not say, "No, wrong." If the student's answer is incorrect, re-ask in a different way to help the student discover the correct answer. This type of teaching helps students maintain a high self-confidence and a more positive attitude toward math.

Step 3: Have the student define a rectangle with the process above.

Step 4: After the student understands what squares and rectangles are and how to describe them, show him how many small squares are contained within a large square. To do this, surround four small squares with a rubber band.

Step 5: Have the student count how many squares are in the large square. Show that each side of the square covers a certain number of square lengths, and each side has the same number of squares. Give one side the label "height", and the other side the label "base". Show that, by multiplying the number of squares in the base by the number in the height, the answer will equal the number of small squares inside the large square surrounded by the rubber band.

Step 6: Now use a rubber band to make a square containing nine boxes. Explain that the base contains three squares and the height contains three squares: 3 x 3 = 9. Show that there are nine small squares. Repeat, using squares of various sizes, until the student gains the concept of area.

Step 7: Repeat Step 6 using rectangles. Be sure the student understands that the base times the height will always be equal to the number of squares enclosed within the rubber-banded shape.

Step 8: Now move on to triangles. This appears tricky because it seems to need a formula, which is not intuitive. When I ask the adults in my audiences if they can remember the formula for the area of a triangle, few can. This is because long ago they may have memorized a formula to get the answer without understanding what the formula meant. After giving them a visual for knowing the area of a triangle, they get the "a-ha" moment and can remember it without difficulty. Encircle a 2x4 rectangle with a rubber band. Show the student that if you cut the rectangle exactly in half horizontally, each side will have the same number of squares. Then show how a vertical cut in the middle of the rectangle would also create the same number of squares on each side. This is usually a simple concept with little or no confusion. Then make a diagonal line cutting the rectangle in half. Ask the student if the two sides are as equal as they were with the horizontal and vertical dividing lines. The answer should be yes. If not, the very young student may not have a fully developed concrete operational understanding. In this case, cut a piece of paper that fits into one of the triangles and have the student move it to the other triangle to show that the paper is the same size and fits on both sides. If this concept is not understood, this procedure is too advanced for the student.

Step 9: Once it is established that the student has developed his concrete operational concepts, then he is ready to learn the area of a triangle. Explain that, since the diagonal line cuts the rectangle into two equal parts, we can determine how many total squares are on each side. Take the area of the rectangle as learned earlier, base times height, and divide it by 2 (or multiply it by ½). Show the student that (b x h)/2 is the same as ½ (b x h). The calculation of a triangle is simply cutting the square or rectangle in half. Show that the diagonal line connects the two corners; one side of the triangle is the base and the other the height.

Step 10: Once the above concepts are understood you are ready to play the game. Encircle an odd shape. Have the student take different colored rubber bands to encircle the squares or rectangles that occupy the shape. Also ask the student to encircle the parts that are only a triangle. He adds the parts together to calculate the area of the odd shape. See Illustration #10.

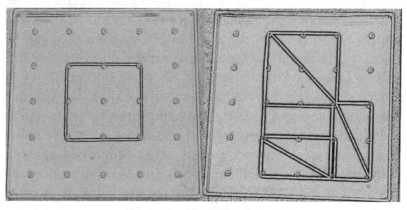

Illustration #10: Geoboards

PARQUETRY BLOCKS

Materials

- Set of parquetry blocks

- 8" x 11" poster board

Procedure:

Step 1: Divide the parquetry blocks into two equal sets, with four triangles, four squares, and four diamonds in each set.

Step 2: The coach and student sit next to each other at a table. The coach makes a design with some of his blocks, ensuring the blocks touch each other. Ask the student to match the design with his blocks. After completing the match ask, "Is your design exactly like mine?" and "Is your design the same distance from you as mine is from me?" If all are matched, repeat with more blocks. If the student notices they are not the same, ask, "How might you change yours so they can match mine exactly?" If the student sees them as the same, but they are not, ask, "How much space is between me and my blocks? Is it larger than, smaller than, or equal to yours?" Work with a variety of leading questions until the student can discover how to make the blocks and the spaces they occupy the same as yours.

Step 3: Once this idea is gained, make designs with the blocks not touching each other, and with a variety of spaces between them.

Step 4: A variation of this activity is to stack some of the blocks.

Step 5: Add *visual memory* to the activity. The coach hides his blocks from the student's view while making a design. When complete, he lets the student view his blocks for about five seconds, then covers them up. Ask the student to make the design from his visual memory. If necessary, use a few blocks at first.

Step 6: Now the coach changes position by sitting directly across from the student. Explain that there is a pretend mirror between the two of you. The coach should make a design with his blocks, and the student should make a mirror image of the design made by the coach. See Illustration #11. The object on right side of the coach's design should match the object on the left side of the student's design.

Step 7: After this concept is gained, add visual memory as in Step 5.

Step 8: While sitting across from each other, take away the pretend mirror and have the student make the design as you see it. The blocks on his right side should be the same as the ones on your right side, and the blocks on his left side should match the ones on your left side.

Step 9: After the Step 8 concept is gained, add visual memory as in Step 5.

	Touching	Not Touching
Side by Side		
Mirror		
No Mirror		

Illustration #11: Parquetry Block Designs

ATTRIBUTE BLOCKS

Materials:

- Set of attribute blocks
- 2 Venn diagrams

Procedure:

Part I:

Step 1: The eyes of students of all ages light up when the attribute blocks are dumped on the table at the beginning of this activity. Everyone seems to want to touch and manipulate them. This creates a positive attitude from the start. Ask the student what he or she sees. When the response is, "Blocks," ask if they are the same or different. The response should be, "Different." Then ask, "How are they different?" Look for the response, "They are different in shape, size, color and thickness." You may need to ask several questions for the student to discover all the different block characteristics. Never give the answer. If the student is stuck identifying one of the characteristics, hold up two blocks that are the same in three ways, but different in one way.

Step 2: Once the student is aware of all four characteristics, hand him the large, thick, yellow square block and ask, "What are the four characteristics of this block?" The response should be, "It is a large, thick, yellow square." Often the student will miss one or more characteristic. If the response is that it is a yellow square, pick up from the pile a small, thin yellow square and ask, "Is your block the same as this one? How is it similar? How is it different?"

Step 3: When the student can correctly and consistently identify the four characteristics of several blocks, ask him for the characteristics in the correct grammatical sequence. That would be, "I have a large, thick, yellow square," not "I have a square, yellow, thick, large."

Part II:

Step 1: Choose one block and place it in front of the student. Ask the student to find another block just like this one, except different in only *one* way. If he chooses one that is different in *more* than one way, ask questions so he can discover how to find a block that is different in only one way. Again, be careful not to tell, but guide him with questions. Never say *no* or *wrong*; just ask a different question. There are many correct answers.

Step 2: If the student picks a piece that is different in one of the four ways, such as color, ask, "Can you find another piece different in only one way, but not different in color?"

Step 3: If he picks one different in size, then ask, "Now can you find one different in one way, but not color or size?"

Step 4: If he now chooses a different shape, ask, "Can you find one different from mine in one way, but not color, size, or shape?" For example, if your piece is a large, thick yellow square, the piece that accurately answers your question is the large, thin yellow square.

Step 5: Ask for a block that is different in two ways.

Step 6: Ask for a block that is different in three ways.

Step 7: Ask for a block that is different in four ways.

Part III:

This part involves playing a game of sets (such as "all red blocks" or "all squares").

Step 1: Place one of the Venn diagrams that comes with the attribute block set on the table in front of the student. Say, "I am thinking of a set. Pick a piece and I will tell you if it belongs." When a block is picked, answer *yes* or *no* as to whether the block belongs. If it does, place it within the Venn diagram. If not, place it just outside the circle. As soon as the student knows the definition of the set, he should define it. If he answers correctly, say, "Yes, that is my set." If not say, "No, that is not my set; choose other pieces to better define my set." The goal is to select as few blocks as possible to determine what your set is.

Step 2: Let the student have a turn and the let the coach discover the set. Begin this part with an easy set, then add more difficult ones.

Step 3: Next, take two Venn diagrams and make two sets. For example, one set might be all red shapes, one set all triangles, and the subset containing attributes that are common to both sets. Have the student decide what the subset is by overlapping the circles and placing the shapes in the area of the subset.

Step 4: Create many variations of sets and subsets. Try the Venn diagrams and discover which are common to all three sets.

MATH STARS

Materials

- Pencil

- Worksheets with the numbers 0 through 9 written in a circle

Procedure:

Step 1: To multiply by a number from 1 through 9, the student will count by that number as he goes around the circle. See Illustration #12. For example, to count by two's, the student places the pencil tip on the zero and draws a line to the number 2, saying "two" out loud. Next, he moves the pencil directly to the number 4, saying "four" out loud. He continues drawing lines to every other number until a pattern emerges. He continues to the number 10 and beyond by going to the last digit of the number. For example, he goes to 0 and says "ten"; the next number ends in 2, he draws a line to the number 2 and says "twelve", and continues following the same pattern. Notice every multiple of this number will stay on the same line of the pattern.

Step 2: Repeat with "3", then "4", then "5" etc.

Step 3: When the student easily and quickly makes it to 100, go backward with each number.

Step 4: For multiplication, the student counts the "number of moves" needed to get to the desired answer. For example, to multiply three times three, you start at zero and move the pencil to three, counting "one" move. Then move the pencil three spaces to the number 6 and count "two" moves. Next move the pencil three spaces to the number 9 and count "three" moves. Thus, the answer to three times three is nine. If multiplying three times four, move the pencil three more spaces to the number 2. This number shows the last digit of the answer: 12.

Notice how each multiple of a different number will create a unique star pattern.

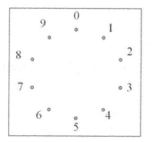 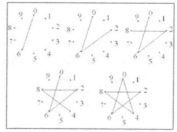

Illustration #12: Math Stars

TROUBLESHOOTING

GRAPH PAPER

It can be difficult to keep the numbers in the correct columns when adding, subtracting or multiplying three or more digits. It is helpful to use graph paper with large spaces to organize the digits. If you do not have graph paper, rotate lined paper 90 degrees and you will have columns to keep the numbers in place.

GAMES

Games that help improve visual thinking skills for math:

- Sudoku puzzles
- Tangoes
- Yahtzee
- Chess
- Battleship
- Perfect Ten Magic Card Trick

SUDOKU

These puzzles are helpful to familiarize the student with the numbers one through nine. As his puzzle-solving skill improves, the student will be building visual memory skills. Begin with very easy puzzles. If still too difficult, fill in some of the numbers to make it easier.

TANGOES

This type of puzzle is more advanced, and can begin to challenge higher-level problem-solving skills. These skills are helpful in upper-level math such as geometry.

YAHTZEE

Yahtzee will familiarize students with number recognition, adding, grouping, and decision-making. This game can be enjoyed by both younger and older students.

CHESS

This game helps to improve strategy, visual memory, and planning skills.

BATTLESHIP

This is good for memory and strategy.

PERFECT TEN MAGIC CARD TRICK

This fun trick helps the student with counting.

SUMMARY

Understanding math concepts requires a student to have a good command of his visual abilities. Helping students gain confidence in their math skills can be accomplished by using the enjoyable activities discussed in this chapter. Relating math to many career choices and to everyday activities will help the student understand why math is important. Math is fun! Gaining math skills will improve your student's future opportunities.

REVIEW

Visual Skills

- Binocularity
- Laterality
- Directionality
- Spatial Organization
- Spatial Orientation
- Visual Closure

- Visual Figure Ground

- Association

- Categorization

Time

- 20 minutes daily for math concepts

- Daily counting steps and stairs, along with games, will develop better math thinking skills

Coaching

- Don't say *no* or *wrong*

- Point out what part of the answer is correct

- Have the student discover which problems need to be fixed

Components and Concepts

- Linear Units

- Addition and Subtraction

- Multiplication and Division

- Fractions

Building Skills

- Counting Steps

- Measuring Objects

- 100 Squares

- Dice Game
- Puzzles

Practice

- Body Movement Multiplication
- Dr. M's Multiplication Math Facts Technique
- Geoboard
- Parquetry Blocks
- Attribute Blocks
- Math Stars

Trouble Shooting

- Graph paper
- Sudoku puzzles
- Tangoes
- Yahtzee
- Chess
- Battleship
- Perfect Ten Magic Card Trick

8

VISUAL SECRETS FOR READING COMPREHENSION

SELF-ESTEEM AND READING ABILITY

The more that you read, the more things you will know. The more that you learn, the more places you'll go.

— Dr. Seuss

Successful reading involves the greatest number of visual skills. Reading ability is affected when students have underdeveloped visual skills; thus, reading is one of the more difficult academic subjects to improve.

There are many opinions on the best way to teach students to be good readers with excellent comprehension. No two students are exactly alike, and one style of teaching does not work for everyone. When a student has been behind his age group in reading for several years, and only one approach has been used over and over with little success, it is no surprise that the student, teacher, and parents are frustrated. Some teaching techniques cause high anxiety, and a big "I hate to read" switch turns on in a student's head every time he is required to read. To overcome this attitude toward reading, the environment, the approach, and the materials used need to be fun, exciting, and easy, so the student can build self-confidence and feel good about reading (and about himself).

VISUAL SKILLS IMPORTANT FOR READING:

Visual Skill	Definition
Saccadic Eye Movement	The ability to accurately shift one's fixation from one target to another
Accommodation	The ability to keep an image in focus when viewed up close
Binocularity	The ability to use the two eyes together so they send the same message to the brain at the same time
Laterality	Correct understanding of one's right and left sides
Directionality	Understanding how you relate to the objects around you and how they relate to each other
Visualization	The ability to see pictures of objects with the eyes closed
Visual Memory	The ability to recall a viewed image over a long period of time
Visual Sequential Memory	The ability to remember the correct sequence of letters and words
Visual Association	The ability to relate common objects and/ or ideas
Visual Categorization	The ability to organize similar objects and concepts
Visual Figure Ground	The ability to stay focused on a figure or an object gazed upon, even when the background information may be confusing and extensive
Visual Identification of Size, Space, and Shape	The ability to recognize and name what is seen

Visual Matching of Size, Space, and Shape	The ability to remember the correct sequence of letters and words
Visual Discrimination of Size, Space, and Shape	The ability to relate common objects and/or ideas

Saccadic Eye Movement: This skill is important for reading because the eyes must move accurately from word to word. If a student's eyes make too large of a shift, he might skip a word. If the shift is too small, he will re-read the same words. These problems interfere with comprehension. Another sign of a problem with saccades is word reversals such as *saw* for *was,* and *god* for *dog.*

Eye Focusing or Accommodation: People will eventually become very familiar with this skill when they approach age 45. Suddenly it will become difficult for them to read text held at near, the text can be blurred, and headaches might result when they push to make their eyes focus. Losing one's ability to focus up close is completely normal after age 45. However, under age 40, students should be able to look at near text for long periods of time without seeing blur. If the text blurs in and out when reading, it becomes difficult to pay attention to the task. If pushed to finish the task, headaches, eye-rubbing, and eyestrain are common results. Eyes are never supposed to hurt when reading. If they hurt or tear up when reading, it is critical to see an optometrist so the issue can be treated. Ignoring these complaints may lead to more severe problems.

EYES ARE NEVER SUPPOSED TO HURT WHEN READING. IF THEY HURT OR TEAR UP WHEN READING, IT IS CRITICAL TO SEE AN OPTOMETRIST SO THE ISSUE CAN BE TREATED.

Eye teaming or binocularity: This is critical for good comprehension, but students without binocularity can become good readers. Mild eye teaming problems usually cause the most trouble, which seems strange. Why would a student with a mild binocular problem have more difficulty than a student with a significant binocular problem? The answer is this: when the eyes are sometimes good at teaming and sometimes poor at it, the print on the page goes in and out of double vision. When the text is double *all* of the time, the brain will usually learn to turn off, or ignore, the input from one eye, which makes the double text easier to ignore. When the brain ignores the input sent from one eye, this is called *suppression*. When a student has a very strong suppression, some of the binocular cells will convert to monocular ones, and the brain becomes better at processing the information. When a small suppression exists, it can create more problems with fatigue, since only 10 percent of the visual cortex cells are processing information.

David Hubel and Torsten Wiesel's breakthrough discoveries about the visual system and visual processing earned them a Nobel Prize in 1981. They discovered that the right eye relates to 10 percent of visual cortex cells, and the left eye to a different 10 percent. The other 80 percent of the visual cortex cells react only when both eyes are used at the same time under a binocular condition.[31] So if the brain suppresses the information from one eye, it shuts down 90 percent of the visual cortex cells needed to process the visual information. In this scenario, the student gets tired very quickly just after he begins to read. Some people use reading as a sleeping pill. Often, these people have a binocular vision problem.

Laterality: Many students use a pneumonic to know which is right and left. Two examples of this are knowing he writes with his right hand, and making the letter *L* with the left index finger and thumb signifying the left hand. Using a pneumonic interferes with the proper development of knowing right and left. Why is this so important for reading?

When laterality is poorly developed, the letters, *b, d, p,* and *q* are often reversed. This makes learning a word confusing and difficult. The letters *b, d,* and *p* are in many words that a new reader is required to learn. To help prevent poor development of laterality, it helps to use the words *right* and *left* when giving directions to a young child.

Do not teach a pneumonic. Instead, educate students to feel the difference between right and left rather than using a thought to recall it. When putting on shoes for the toddler, say, "This is your right shoe going on your right foot." When the child practices balancing, he learns that he has a center and two different sides. So, lots of outside balancing activities help to develop this skill. An optometrist can perform a specific test called the Piaget Left/Right Awareness Test to check laterality issues. If not well developed by age seven, Optometric Vision Therapy (OVT) can be used to treat this problem.

Directionality: This is important for understanding the meaning of sentences that incorporate directional words such as *up, down, in, out, over, under, north, south, east,* and *west.* When a student has directional confusion, he can have difficulty understanding these words when they are used for instruction. Directional words are used in many instructions given to students, both verbally and written. When reading directional words, the student must think about what the words mean before being able to understand what is being asked. The OVT used for laterality development can also be helpful for directionality understanding.

Visualization or Visual Imagery: Visualization is the ability to see an image in one's mind of something recently viewed. Some refer to this as Visual Imagery. This skill is extremely important for young students because it helps them remember words that are newly learned or sounded out. Good visualizers can read a book as if they are watching a movie. Sub-vocalization or auditory reassurance occurs when saying the words in one's head while reading. This can interfere with visualization, and can make the student a slower reader.

Visual Memory: When a student has poor ability to visualize and no short-term visual memory, he has difficulty remembering a word he sees on page 3 that he had just sounded out on page 1. Clinically, I have noticed that teaching a student to visualize is fairly easy up until about age 12. After age 12, the student's habit of not being able to make a visual picture is more embedded. A student who sees black in his mind's eye instead of an image or a picture must use his non-visual memory to recall the details of information being read. See Chapter 5 on spelling to help a small child develop visualization skills by telling descriptive stories.

Visual Sequential Memory: This is good for understanding what is seen, and for good comprehension. Students with poor Visual Sequential Memory can have difficulty with grammar rules and spelling.

Visual Association: This skill is important for comprehension.

Visual Categorization: This is important for higher levels of comprehension.

Visual Figure Ground: The smaller the print and the closer the words are to each other, the higher the level of figure ground discrimination required. Problems with figure ground can be identified when the student has lost his place when reading, and he cannot find it again because all of the words around it create a confusing background. Toddler activities such as puzzle making, bird watching, and coloring can help develop good figure ground skills.

Visual Identification of Size, Space, and Shape: Difficulty with this skill creates problems with letter and word recognition.

*Visual Matching of Size, Space, and Shape***:** The words *mountain* and *mountains* are very similar in appearance and meaning. Knowing that the letter *s* at the end of the word indicates more than one is important for understanding what is being read.

Visual Discrimination of Size, Space, and Shape: This is helpful when trying to differentiate and read words that are similar, such as *the* and *then*. The This-That-Then Confusion Technique described below helps overcome issues with visual discrimination.

We have defined many visual skills important for reading. It is clear that when a visual problem exists, the student will have more difficulty learning to read. Once these visual skills are correctly developed, it will be easier for the student to enjoy reading and to be successful at it. When poor reading habits and a negative psychological attitude toward reading are strongly embedded, it may be difficult for the student to incorporate these new visual skills.

The following ideas demonstrate how to change these habits so the student with well-developed visual skills can improve his reading skills. Remember, it is critical to start these procedures after the student has the visual skills of tracking, eye teaming, figure ground and visualization assessed by a licensed optometrist. If the visual skills are not present or are underdeveloped, the student and the coaches will continue to be frustrated.

> IT IS CRITICAL TO START THESE PROCEDURES AFTER THE STUDENT HAS THE VISUAL SKILLS NEEDED TO PERFORM READING. IF THE VISUAL SKILLS ARE NOT PRESENT OR ARE UNDERDEVELOPED, THE STUDENT AND THE COACHES WILL CONTINUE TO BE FRUSTRATED.

TIME

Work on the Building Reading Skills techniques for ten to fifteen minutes to encourage students to be ready to read. With gentle coaching, spend fifteen minutes daily on silent reading.

COACHING

To develop comprehension, it is critical that the student's eye-brain process of the information being read is not interrupted or diverted. Making the student stop and sound out unknown words puts the eye-brain process on hold. The student may entirely forget what has been read.

Have the student point to a word that he doesn't know and simply tell him what it is. Do not make him sound it out. Ask the student if he understands what the word means. If he doesn't, define it for him. If the student can use the word correctly in a sentence, then usually the word will be retained for quicker recall the next time it is encountered.

Randomly point to five words in the text. If the student does not know the words, the level of reading is too difficult. Either reduce the reading level, or build the student's vocabulary for words that will be encountered in the reading material. Techniques for building vocabulary are described below in the Word Recognition Technique.

Reading was so difficult.

Listening to Laney read was almost painful. She had to sound out every word, she did not use facial expressions, and reading a paragraph took a long time. Homework time was becoming stressful for the family and often ended in tears.

It was determined that Laney had multiple visual problems that were stopping her from learning to read with ease. Laney had uncorrected 20/20 eyesight, but had double vision and difficulty with eye movements when reading. Besides poor visual motor skills, Laney also had undeveloped laterality, visualization, visual memory and figure ground skills. After finishing an optometric vision therapy program, Laney's visual skills improved.

Laney was a bright child but her former habits prevented her from using her newly-developed visual skills for reading. She, her optometrist and her parents worked on the Visual Secrets for Reading and she began to improve. It wasn't until she found a book about a horse, which she loved and read from cover to cover, that she began to enjoy reading. Fortunately, the book was a series of several books and as soon as she finished one, she wanted to read the next one. After reading three of these books for fun, her reading skills improved markedly. Today she is in college majoring in English.

READING COMPONENTS

- Reading materials
- Proper lighting
- Anti-reflective coating lenses
- Visor
- Yummy beverage
- Music
- Font
- Print size
- Bold print

READING MATERIALS

First, begin with interesting reading materials, which may be different for young female students versus young male students. Little girls tend to enjoy fiction books, therefore cute animals or fantasy topics are more interesting. Little boys tend to like non-fiction books, humor, or stories with topics that many women may find gross. Examples of books boys may be more attracted to include *Captain Underpants* or books about poisonous frogs. Sometimes it is better if dad, big brother or a male role model helps select reading materials for boys rather than the female teacher or mom making the selection. It is important to know the student's interest and find a book about that subject.

Years ago I had a fourth-grade boy who had completed his Optometric Vision Therapy program but still disliked reading, even though he had been able to develop the visual skills needed for reading. When I asked him what he would enjoy reading, his answer was, "Barracuda cars." I thought, *Oh, no! How will we ever find a book on what he enjoys?* However, much to mom's credit, she searched everywhere to find a book about Barracuda cars. He loved the book and read it cover to cover, over and over again. When he returned for a progress evaluation, his mom stated that he now enjoyed reading and was doing very well with required reading assignments, too. Sometimes it just takes one book to create the *a-ha* response, or the "I've got it!" I have seen this happen at all ages.

Changing the desire to read can happen at any age. A very bright young man who did well in school disliked reading and never read for pleasure. His girlfriend wrote a novel and asked him to read it. His desire to please his girlfriend led him to read it, and he became interested in the story. After reading her book, he began to enjoy reading for pleasure. This type of interested focus helped him enjoy the experience of reading the story. Her novel had created curiosity about the plot, and he developed a positive attitude while reading the story. For some students, it can take reading up to four books with the "I want to know what happens" attitude before the joy of reading takes hold and becomes automatic.

It is extremely important for a child to like what he is reading in order to create a desire to know the end of the story. Curiosity, interest and fun overcome the negative response to reading. Dull and boring topics reinforce the feeling that reading is horrible and should be avoided whenever possible. Students having difficulty learning to read are repeatedly given basic, non-interesting, easy to read material that increases the boredom. To avoid a *bored, forced* reading situation, you might want to create a more positive situation with the following suggestions:

PROPER LIGHTING

The healthiest light is sunlight or candlelight, followed by full-spectrum incandescent light, then halogen light, then light emitting diode (LED), then compact fluorescent light (CFL). Fluorescent is the most common form of lighting in schools;

however, it can be very irritating for a reader. Symptoms that could be related to fluorescent lighting are:

- Eyestrain
- Light sensitivity
- Reduced reading proficiency[32]
- Increase in eye disease[33]
- Mental and physical fatigue [3]
- Reduced alertness [3]
- Difficulty sleeping [3]
- Headache or migraine[34]
- Over activity [4]
- Muscle tension [3]

ANTI-REFLECTIVE COATING

Special reading lenses with specific anti-reflective coatings can help students stay focused while reading. Optometrists specializing in Optometric Vision Therapy have unique training to prescribe a "boost" lens for reading and computer work that give students added support while performing near tasks such as reading, writing, or working on digital devices.

VISOR

A visor or a hat with a brim can offset the effects of fluorescent lighting when it is impossible to avoid. The brim reduces the amount of light that the visual system is processing, which allows the eyes to have an easier time sending the reading message to the brain. An optometrist can write a prescription to allow your student to wear a hat in class if this is an issue.

YUMMY BEVERAGE

Enjoyable beverages such as hot cocoa or coffee enhance the reading experience. Coffee shops have figured this out. Often these cozy places have comfy chairs with rows of interesting reading materials. Enjoying a tasty, "cozy" beverage while reading an interesting book will make the experience even better. Set up an area in the home that can simulate this type of a cozy atmosphere and be ready with the student's favorite warm beverage.

MUSIC

> LISTENING TO MUSIC CAN IMPROVE READING FOCUS. SELF-SELECTED, ENJOYABLE, SOFT, RELAXING BACKGROUND MUSIC WITHOUT WORDS CAN CREATE A MORE POSITIVE ENVIRONMENT DURING READING ACTIVITIES.

Listening to music can improve reading focus. Self-selected, enjoyable, soft, relaxing background music without words can create a more positive environment during reading activities. Ask your student how certain music makes him feel. Words such as *relaxed, quiet,* and *comfortable* indicate you have the right selection, whereas words such as *mad, anxious,* and *stressed* would not normally be helpful.[35]

FONT

Be aware of the font because the type used can be critical to efficient reading. Some fonts have serifs and some do not. Serif fonts, such as Times New Roman, can be defined as having "feet" added to letters. These feet, tails, flourishes, and curves (serifs) simulate how we write by hand. They trick our brain to seeing it as handwriting.[36]

The fonts that don't have these features, such as Helvetica and Arial, are called sans-serif (without serifs) fonts. Read the two paragraphs in Illustration #13. The first is in Times New Roman font, and the second is in Arial font.

Times New Roman Font

By understanding the complexity of vision and having the love of inspiring and helping patients improve their lives, Dr. Brenda Montecalvo teaches her readers how to use vision more efficiently. The methods in *Visual Secrets for School Success* provide the reader with the most valuable currency available on earth: *time*. We have only a limited amount of time, and we desire to have more quality time with those who are the most important to us. Inefficient learners may read slower, misspell words, have poor math skills, or have difficulty writing, which takes more time to get most jobs done. Stress increases when there is little time for a high-quality life. When people can be more efficient at learning their stress is reduced, they feel better about who they are and what they can do. They are more in control of their lives. They are empowered. They *win* at life.

Arial Font

By understanding the complexity of vision and having the love of inspiring and helping patients improve their lives, Dr. Brenda Montecalvo teaches her readers how to use vision more efficiently. The methods in *Visual Secrets for School Success* provide the reader with the most valuable currency available on earth: *time*. We have only a limited amount of time, and we desire to have more quality time with those who are the most important to us. Inefficient learners may read slower, misspell words, have poor math skills, or have difficulty writing, which takes more time to get most jobs done. Stress increases when there is little time for a high quality life. When people can be more efficient at learning their stress is reduced, they feel better about who they are and what they can do. They are more in control of their lives. They are empowered. They *win* at life.

Illustration #13: Two Types of Fonts

Sarah Morrison and Jan Noyes, of the University of Bristol, showed that Times New Roman is the best typeface for reading any document. Readers speed through material with its simple letters. Times New Roman has letters that are easier to recognize because they are associated with handwritten letters. [36, 38]

The brain also has a variety of orientation cells that recognize parts of objects. Some cells recognize horizontal lines, some recognize vertical lines, and some recognize diagonal lines. Serif fonts have more of all of these lines. This gives the brain more identification clues, which makes it easier to recognize the combination of letters and turn it into meaning. A sans-serif font, while looking cleaner, gives less information for recognition, thus taking a longer time for the brain to process and convert into understanding.

PRINT SIZE

Determine if enlarged print is helpful. When a student is beginning to read, the print size is large. Each year, the print size shrinks. This continues to occur until about fifth or sixth grade. If the student has visual-motor problems in the areas of tracking, focusing, or eye teaming, decreased print size exacerbates these problems. A student with these problems can still have 20/20 visual acuity, but poor vision. Repairing these problems with an Optometric Vision Therapy program is recommended. Until the problems are resolved, the student will continue to struggle to be a successful reader. In these cases, try to enlarge the font size of the required reading as much as possible so the student does not struggle because of an uncorrected visual motor skill problem.

To determine the best font size for easy reading, the optometrist measures the student's efficiency of reading sentences containing different font sizes, from large print to small. This evaluation can be done silently by watching the student's eyes while reading. When the student's eyes look at the same word more than once, or appear to skip a word or line, that tells the optometrist the font size is too small. Once the best size is determined, use that size font when building reading skills.

BOLD PRINT

Bold print and background contrast can improve the eye-brain process. Besides enlarging the print, making it bold gives better contrast against the white background. Boldface font enhances identification, making reading easier. There is the occasional student for whom a sharp contrast will reduce his ability to focus on the words and cause eyestrain. When this is the case, the background may need to be less white, or buff color.

Printing words on bold, brightly colored paper can be very disruptive and is never recommended. Determine what is best for the student by varying the font, bold print and background colors. Ask the student which one feels better, both in his head and in his eyes. Use the one the student chooses until his visual system is ready to read with any type of contrast.

BUILDING SKILLS

- Word Recognition
- This-That-Then Confusion Technique
- Expressive Reading
- New Word Recognition
- Constructing Sentences

WORD RECOGNITION

Have the student do word recognition activities. It is important to build a student's vocabulary so there is little need to sound out words when reading. Having to sound out each word interrupts the flow of thought and reduces comprehension. To accomplish a bigger vocabulary, first choose a specific subject. Make a list of 25 words related to that subject, such as volcanoes. The list may look like this: *volcano, molten, rock, stratovolcano, shield, cinder, dormant, active, eruption, lava, mountain, earth, core, rupture, ash, crust, tectonic plate, mantle, hot, soft, gasses, vent, fragments, surface, Alaska, California, Mexico, Hawaii, Washington.* Access a news story about volcanoes and show the student pictures of an eruption.

Materials:

- Paragraphs at different reading levels

Procedure:

Part I:

Step 1: Ask, "Do you know what lava is?" Let the student attempt to define the word. If accurate, have him use the word *lava* in a sentence. Have him say the word softly, then very loudly.

Step 2: Now he is ready to see what the word looks like. Show him the word embedded in a paragraph. Have him pronounce it while looking at it.

Step 3: Next, take the paragraph away momentarily, then show it again to see if he can find the word *lava*. If *lava* is used more than once in the paragraph, ask him to see if he can determine how many times it is used.

Step 4: Repeat this procedure with other difficult words in the paragraph. It may sound tedious, but once the student has an image or picture in his mind of what the written word represents, he is more likely to easily recall it, know it, and not need to sound it out when he sees it next time.

This system allows the student to build something called the *visual dictionary,* which is in the mid-temporal area of the brain. Research shows that this area of the brain is much larger for good readers than it is for poor readers.[37] When my patients are taught this method, I end the session by showing them that they just learned some really big words that are rated as seventh-grade words. I ask them if they are in seventh grade, and they reply *no*. (They are usually in first, second, third, or fourth grade, reading below grade level.) After successfully learning these difficult words, they then read a sentence from the same paragraph that has the words in it. Their success at this gives them tremendous self-confidence and the belief that they really can read challenging material. I explain that many students in their grade cannot read the words they just read. Their faces reflect the pride they gain in themselves once they understand they are doing something very advanced. This is very rewarding for all involved.

> WORD RECOGNITION ALLOWS THE STUDENT TO BUILD SOMETHING CALLED THE *VISUAL DICTIONARY,* WHICH IS IN THE MID-TEMPORAL AREA OF THE BRAIN. RESEARCH SHOWS THAT THIS AREA OF THE BRAIN IS MUCH LARGER IN GOOD READERS THAN IT IS IN POOR READERS.

Part II: Practice the new words.

Step 1: Once a student has learned 20 new words, type them several times randomly in bold, 14-point Times New Roman font. Have the student read the words quickly without hesitation. Time him on how long it takes. Ask him to read them again to see if he can beat his time. Give a reward if he does. (Yes, gold stars still work for most students).

Step 2: Turn the paper upside down and see if he can still read the words. Time him to see if he can read them as fast upside down as he can right side up. This will build automaticity of knowing the words every time he sees them in a text.

THIS-THAT-THEN CONFUSION TECHNIQUE

Students who have difficulty reading and comprehending can confuse similarly spelled words such as *this, them, that, there, then*, etc. Once the brain creates confusion between two or more words and mixes them up, the confusion is reinforced. When seeing one of the two words, the brain thinks, *I wonder which one it is. I'm not sure. I know it is one of these two words.* To stop the confusion, the brain needs to override it with accurate, first-time recall of the word. Repetition is the key to creating automatic recognition. The eye-brain process must recall the word accurately at least 15 times to override the confusion between two words.

Materials

- This-That-Then Chart, See Illustration #14

Procedure:

Step 1: For the This-That-Then Confusion Technique, make a list of all the similar-sounding and similar-looking words. Put all the *th* sight words on one list, and all the *wh* sight words on a different list.

Step 2: Take one list and type out a chart using the words repeatedly and randomly. See Illustration #14. Be sure the words are in large font, bold, lower case Times New Roman font.

Step 3: Have the student call out the words as rapidly as possible. When a word is misspoken, point back and forth between the two miscalled words until they are called out accurately. An example is, "This, that, this, that, this, that," if there is no miscalling. When the student is beginning to figure out correct calling, you may hear "This, that . . . tha-this . . . that . . . tha-a . . . is." This can be frustrating for the student, so make it fun with rewards, cheering and smiles. *Never* say, "No, you are wrong." Simply point to the word until it is correctly called. Or say, "Almost!" Let the student discover how to catch and fix an error. It is very important to keep this positive and make it feel like a game. Laughter is good, too. The goal is to call each word quickly and accurately with no hesitation, creating automatic recall.

this	that	them	then	their
there	then	that	their	this
that	this	their	there	them
then	them	that	this	there
them	this	then	that	their

Illustration #14: This-That-Then Chart

EXPRESSIVE READING

Teaching expressive reading requires the student to read out loud. While reading out loud may not be practical, it can be taught so the student can experience success in school. When reading aloud in the classroom, the teacher and the other students hear the mistakes. This can be very embarrassing and lead to an even greater dislike of reading. For this reason, it is important to be able to read aloud well. It is important to note: reading out loud may not have a positive impact on silent reading with good comprehension.

Do you remember when you were in kindergarten, before you could read? The teacher would gather all the children in a circle and read to them. She would glance at the book, but look around at the children when telling the story. The book was usually held up so everyone could see the pictures. This is an expressive reading environment.

Begin by choosing reading material that is slightly below the student's reading ability. The goal is to read without having to sound out a word, so it is important for the student to visually recognize all of the words with quick recall. Have the student take a good look at the first few words, then look up at the person to whom he is reading. The student only says the words when looking up. He fixates the next set of words to be read then looks up and says the words. It is also critical that he listens to what he is saying so that he can use the correct expression that relates to the words being read. Looking at oneself in the mirror can substitute if the student does not want to look at the coach. This is referred to as reading to the mirror.

NEW WORD RECOGNITION

How many children can read the signs for McDonald's, Walmart, or Target at age two? Almost all children can, unless they have not experienced regular visits to these places. How many two-year-olds have been taught phonetics? Not too many, yet based on this observation it is possible to learn to read words without phonetics. Phonetics makes learning to read easier for many students, but not for all students. The young student who is stuck and not learning any words needs to build confidence by increasing his vocabulary. Pushing sight words first is much more difficult for this type of student. Adults think a small three-letter word such as *the*, should be easy to learn. But what does *the* mean to a new reader? What visual picture is related to *the*? Compared to McDonald's, *the* is very boring, not interesting, and creates no curiosity. So instead of pushing the sight words, maybe it would be better to build the noun and verb groups first, then use the sight words when trying to connect these words to make a sentence.

Materials:

- Signs of objects in home
- Stopwatch
- Large surface area, such as a dining room table

Procedure:

Step 1: Make ten signs to be placed on ten objects in the home. Let the student choose the objects. The signs should be large, 48-point Times New Roman font, bold, and lower case. The signs stay on the objects for three days.

Step 2: The student is told that, in three days, the signs will be removed.

Step 3: The student looks at the signs daily. He should understand that after the third day he will put the signs back on the correct objects while he is timed with a stop watch. Make sure the student understands it will be a game to find out how many signs he can place correctly, and how quickly he can do so.

Step 4: On the third day, remove all of the signs and have the student place them back on the objects. Repeat several times. See if he can reduce the time it takes to put the signs back.

Step 5: After he is 100 percent correct, take the signs and stack them in a pile face down. Have him flip them over and say each word. Time him. Repeat and see if he can beat his time. Then turn the words upside down and repeat flipping them over and saying them. The goal is to say each word as quickly upside down as right side up. Next, label ten different objects and repeat the above procedure, except when stacking the signs use all of the learned words. Try to build up the stack of words to 100 words.

CONSTRUCTING SENTENCES

Procedure:

Step 1: Sentences require more than just nouns. Have the student take the stack of words from the word recognition activity, and on a large surface (like the dining room table) ask him to make a sentence.

Step 2: When the student needs a verb or a sight word, make a sign for those words. The table and chairs are in the dining room. The underlined words are already learned, so he would need to make signs for the words *the*, *and*, *are*, and *in* to complete the sentence. Now the sight words have some meaning and connection. Also, there is more interest in using and learning them. Repeat this activity using several sentences.

Step 3: After the student recognizes new verbs and sight words, have him do the "flip and time" activity as described above. Time him both upside down and right side up. Fast recall ensures better automaticity in knowing the words. Later on, this will help with faster reading while achieving excellent comprehension.

PRACTICE

- Silent Reading
- Pre-Selected Words
- Pre-Ask Questions

SILENT READING

> ENCOURAGE SILENT READING INSTEAD OF READING ALOUD. SILENT READING IS FASTER, WITH IMPROVED COMPREHENSION.

Encourage silent reading instead of reading aloud.[38] Silent reading is faster, with improved comprehension. In an attempt to teach reading, there is a strong push in elementary grades for students to read every word out loud. The evidence suggests that very good readers do not read every word, and when they are asked to read out loud, they must work hard to slow down.

Some students are assigned to read out loud 20 minutes each night. I often ask parents if they have ever read out loud every word, very fast, for 20 minutes. Few have. I also ask, "When, as adults, are we required to read like this?" Never. As adults, when asked to read out loud, the best way to do it is to read slowly with lots of expression in order to hold the audience's attention. Examples of this are narrating a play or reading in a group when studying a specific text (as in a Bible study).

Reading out loud is fine sometimes, but silent reading is more important to develop reading skills. What indicates to you that a student is remembering what he is reading? Simple: ask questions about the text.

Have the student read a paragraph. If he gets to a word that he does not know, he points to it and you, the coach, tell him the word. This support prevents disruption of the flow of thought while reading. Phonetically sounding out words can be saved for another vocabulary learning time. Ask a general question about who the characters are or what the paragraph is about. Ask specific, detailed questions about the reading material. These questions indicate the depth of understanding. Also, the student's correct responses indicate the material he read is registered in the thinking eye-brain process.

PRE-SELECTED WORDS

Pre-select unrelated words from the reading material. Pre-read a chapter that the student will read. Choose five words that are found in the chapter. It is okay if they do not appear to relate to each other. Ask the student to determine how the words may relate prior to reading the chapter. Can he make up a story using the five words? Then have him read the chapter and indicate how the words *actually* relate to each other. This helps to improve interest and curiosity while reading.

PRE-ASK QUESTIONS

Create curiosity with pre-reading and pre-asked questions.

Choose an interesting subject for the student to read, one that creates curiosity. If the student is turned off by volcanoes, for example, don't pick volcanoes. Try to find a subject related to a sport or hobby the student enjoys. Pre-read the first chapter. Create five questions about the chapter. Ask the student the questions before he reads the chapter. Have the student attempt to answer the questions even though he has not done the reading required to answer the questions. Next, have him read the chapter and then re-ask the exact same questions. Let him discover if his answers were correct or not. The curiosity about the real answers helps increase interest while reading.

TROUBLESHOOTING

Students who have been forced to read can have a very negative attitude toward reading even when they have all the tools to be a good reader. Helping the student get over the negative internal talk is important so reading can be fun. These techniques create a more positive situation to turn on the eye-brain process when beginning to read a text.

LAP READING

Procedure

Step 1: Coaches, put down the cell phone, forget that dinner is not made, and do not allow for any interruptions from spouse or siblings.

Step 2: Select a comfortable chair that allows for good posture. For smaller students, have them sit on the coach's lap while reading. When students are too big to fit on the coach's lap, sit next to them while reading. The arms of the coach and student should be touching. This gives a very positive message.

Students will feel connected because the coach is fully engaged. For the *entire* time students are reading, they know they have the coach's fullest attention. Do not say much; just be there. This gives the student a positive sense of connection before beginning to read.

Step 3: If the student gets to a word of which he knows the meaning when hearing it spoken, but doesn't know it when seeing it in print, have him point to the word. The coach says the word, but the student does not say the word. After the student hears it, he should continue reading. This prevents disruption of the flow of reading.

Step 4: If the student gets to a word of which he doesn't know the meaning when hearing it spoken or seeing it in print, he should ask the coach to define and describe it. Once defined, have the student reread the sentence, instead of just continuing on, to be sure there is comprehension.

READING UPSIDE DOWN

Phonetics has been over-emphasized for several years to teach poor readers to read. Some students can get "stuck" in phonetic reading and have difficulty converting to efficient silent reading. When reading out loud, many or all words are sounded out. When trying to read silently, the lips will be moving. This is referred to as "lip reading." With a bright student, this habit can be difficult to break. For these students, have them read while holding the book upside-down. Use reading material about two grade levels below their level. Most students enjoy the challenge, and are surprised that it can be done. This procedure can turn the "I hate to read" attitude into "I wonder if I can do this?"

I had a patient who was in sixth grade. He had completed a full program of Optometric Vision Therapy, but was not converting his new skills into better reading ability. He had an IQ of about 130, which is very high. I had him read upside down for ten minutes a day. In four weeks, his reading took off and he began to enjoy reading. This had a very positive impact on his success in all subjects. Today he is a professor of engineering.

BIG WORDS

Building confidence is often achieved by showing students they can actually read larger, more advanced words. Pick a subject the student enjoys. Find some twelfth-grade words related to the subject, and use the Word Recognition Technique described above. Emphasize that the student is probably reading words no one in his class knows how to read.

SUMMARY

Reading is one of the more difficult skills to improve due to the complexity and the variety of visual skills needed to do it well. Self-esteem, motivation, and confidence have been linked to reading skills. The aforementioned activities are for a variety of reading levels. Some are for new readers, some are for readers with bad habits, and some are designed to improve comprehension for all readers. The goal is for students to begin reading for fun and ultimately to enjoy reading. When a student enjoys reading, he is more likely to feel better about himself. When mom says, "Put that book down, it's time to eat," and the student replies, "Just let me finish this chapter," a reader has been born.

REVIEW

Visual Skills

- Saccades (Eye Movements)

- Accommodation (Eye Focusing)

- Binocularity (Eye Teaming)

- Laterality
- Directionality
- Visualization
- Visual Memory
- Visual Sequential Memory
- Visual Association
- Visual Categorization
- Visual Figure Ground
- Visual Identification of Size, Space, and Shape
- Visual Matching of Size, Space, and Shape
- Visual Discrimination of Size, Space, and Shape

Time

- 10-15 minutes daily to work on building reading skills
- 15 minutes of daily silent reading with gentle coaching

Coaching

- Minimize interruptions and use more positives, with an encouraging style of coaching
- Allow the student to discover and ask for help instead of pointing out mistakes

Components

- Reading materials
- Proper lighting

- Anti-reflective coating
- Visor
- Yummy beverage
- Music
- Font
- Print size
- Bold print

Building Skills

- Word Recognition
- This-That-Then Confusion Technique
- Expressive Reading
- New Word Recognition
- Constructing Sentences

Practice

- Silent Reading
- Pre-Selected Words
- Pre-Ask Questions

Trouble Shooting

- Lap Reading
- Upside Down Reading
- Big Words

PART III

THE TREASURE: TIME TO EXCEL

9

TAKING ADVANTAGE OF SPARE TIME IN SCHOOL

TIME SHOULD NOT BE WASTED

Time = Life. Therefore, waste your time and waste your life,
or master your time and master your life.

— Alan Lakein

Managing time is a key to surpassing one's expectations for successful learning. Use time efficiently by learning the *Visual Secrets for School Success.*

Time. Why talk about time? Time is finite for each individual living on earth. Once it is gone, you cannot get it back. One can never make more time. No money on earth can buy even one extra second of time, and a day cannot be made longer. Each person has only a certain amount of time on this earth, so one shouldn't waste a second of time.

If a task can be done well in less time, then do it. In addition to helping students become more successful, *Visual Secrets for School Success* was written to help students have more quality time. When students learn how to complete assignments accurately and quickly, they will have time to do other important activities. When students have time to do things they enjoy, they are happier, they feel better about themselves, and they are ready to make a difference in other people's lives.

WHEN STUDENTS LEARN HOW TO COMPETE ASSIGNMENTS ACCURATELY AND QUICKLY, THEY WILL HAVE TIME TO DO OTHER IMPORTANT ACTIVITIES.

The activities discussed in Chapters 4 through 8 are designed to teach students how to accomplish assignments more quickly and still get great grades.

VISUAL SKILLS NEEDED FOR TIME MANAGEMENT:

Visual Skill	Definition
Binocularity	The ability to use the two eyes together so they send the same message to the brain at the same time
Accommodation	The ability to keep an image in focus when viewed up close
Temporal Localization	How long it takes for an action to occur
Temporal Organization	The synchrony between the eye-brain process and the environment for maintaining the internal clock system
Temporal Orientation	The eye-brain process of comparing events as they relate to when they happen
Visualization	The ability to see pictures with the eyes closed
Visual Memory	The ability to recall a viewed image over an extended period of time

Binocularity: When a student has either over-convergence or under-convergence, it can affect his ability to judge time. A student with an over-convergent visual posture tends to underestimate how much time an activity might take. The student with an under-convergence would think they have more time than they need to get the task completed.

Accommodation: The ability to hold focus on a target relates to time. It helps the convergence system accurately and consistently judge where things are.

Temporal Localization: As objects move through space, it is important to be able to judge their locations in space, and the times they will be at those locations. Knowing where an object is and where it is going helps students determine how much time it will take for the object to arrive at its destination. As an example, if a student sees how slowly or quickly a door is closing, he can determine how much time he has to walk through the doorway to avoid being hit by the door.

Temporal Organization: The internal clock helps the student judge how long it takes to complete an assignment.

Temporal Orientation: This is helpful for being able to build time-telling and understanding of seasonal change skills.

Visualization: Being able to estimate the amount of space occupied by time is aided by being able to see that space.

Visual Memory: It is easier to remember how long a task takes if there is good ability to have a visual memory of the previous experience.

TIME

Spend ten to fifteen minutes daily completing the activities. Throughout the day, make references to time so the students begin to automatically think about time and how it relates to all the activities in which they are participating.

COACHING

Talk about time throughout the day. Ask the student what time it is. Be positive and ask questions when the response is not correct. Have a clock near the student's bed and refer to it upon waking and going to sleep.

COMPONENTS

- Wrist Watch
- Bedside Alarm Clock
- Stopwatch
- Digital Devices

WRIST WATCH

Have students wear a wristwatch with a second hand. Encourage them to play the Time Estimation Game explained under the Practice section in this chapter.

BEDSIDE ALARM CLOCK

Have a clock near the student's bed and refer to it upon waking and going to sleep. If the clock also has a wake-up light, you can set it to match the sunrise and sunset. This type of clock is called a "Wake-Up Light Alarm Clock," and it helps the natural circadian rhythm of the eye-brain process and sets the student's internal clock. Circadian rhythms are the biological processes that are affected by light and darkness.

STOPWATCH

Step 1: The stopwatch can be used for any of the Visual Secret Techniques in Chapters 4 through 8 when timing is needed.

Step 2: Have the student estimate how long it will take him to do a certain task. Use easy tasks at first, such as feeding the dog. Then move to more complicated ones like, "How long do you think it will take to clean your room?"

Step 3: When the student competes the task in the correctly estimated time, then he should receive an award. In this activity, it is preferred to only reward for results close to the estimated time. More points can be given for completion within one minute, less for five minutes, and so on.

DIGITAL DEVICES

Say no to excessive digital device use. If a student decides that spending all day playing video games is his priority, then he will need to be guided by showing him how that will interfere with reaching his life goals. Ask if playing the game is his number-one priority.

> SAY NO TO EXCESSIVE DIGITAL DEVICE USE. CHILDREN WHO SPEND TWO OR MORE HOURS A DAY LOOKING AT SCREENS ARE FOUND TO HAVE LOWER SCORES ON TESTS THAT FOCUS ON THINKING AND LANGUAGE SKILLS.

Today, children spend way too much time exposed to digital devices, and research is showing how this hurts their brain processing. Children who spend two or more hours a day looking at screens are found to have lower scores on tests that focus on thinking and language skills.[39] The first brain scans from The ABCD Study have been analyzed, and researchers have concluded that children who spend more than seven hours a day on screens experience "premature thinning of the cortex," according to Gayla Dowling.[40]

Understanding addiction to television and digital devices helps emphasize to students and their parents the importance of minimizing use of these devices. Overuse of digital devices will not make them better students, more efficient readers or get them into a quality college or trade school. It is easier to strictly minimize their use when students are young than it is to take the devices away later. When the use of digital devices is minimal, children are happier and they argue less frequently with their siblings and parents.

—◦◦◦—

When my kids were young and at home with a babysitter, I always mandated no screen time. If the sun was shining, I preferred they be playing outside. When I came home after work I could always tell when my "screen time rule" was not being followed based on how well my kids got along with each other. It would take about two weeks to undo the negative effects of excessive screen time. In addition to taking up valuable time, lots of screen activity teaches the brain to be in a sleep-like state. Lengthy digital device viewing reinforces poor posture, interferes with language development, and makes students consider reading a boring activity. I knew I had won the screen-time battle with my kids when they preferred reading a book to watching a program on the television.

BUILDING SKILLS

Students need to change how they think about work that is assigned in class. Students who use *Visual Secrets for School Success* read faster, think quicker, and compose essays with ease. They will be able to complete in-class assignments in a shorter period of time than the other students. After students complete in-class assignments, they should then start working on their homework. A goal should be for the students to take no books home at the end of the day by completing all homework assignments before the last bell rings. If there is a study hall, they shouldn't waste time chatting or looking out the window, but should work on their homework assignments. Encourage your students to get to the study hall location quickly and get started right away on assignments.

PRACTICE:

TIME ESTIMATION

Materials:

- Stopwatch

Procedure:

Step 1: Explain that with eyes closed students are to estimate how long 10 seconds lasts without counting in their heads.

Step 2: Have the student close his eyes and be prepared to raise his hand when the 10-second time has ended.

Step 3: Say, "Start," and begin the stopwatch. When the student raises his hand, stop the watch.

Step 4: Show the student the watch and let him discover how close to estimating the 10 seconds he was.

Step 5: Repeat until the student is correct every time.

Step 6: Increase time to 15 seconds and repeat Steps 2 through 6. Continue to increase time until the student can accurately judge one minute of time.

Step 7: Vary the time estimated. Do 5 seconds, then 45, then 20, etc.

SPACE ESTIMATION

Materials:

- Chair

- Bright red object that can be moved easily. One possible example might be a red toy that can easily be picked up with one hand.

Procedure:

Step 1: Explain that the object will be placed a few feet away from the student. Begin at approximately five feet. The student will look at the space between himself and the object, and estimate how many normal steps he thinks it will take for him to reach the object. Discourage counting in the head while performing the next step.

Step 2: Have the student walk to the object and pick it up. Ask the student how close he was to his estimate. Encourage the student to use the same size steps that he would normally use while walking. Repeat with varying distances. The further away the object is placed, the more difficult the task will be.

Step 3: Place a chair between the student and the object. Repeat Step 2. Note: Be sure the student moves around the chair without hitting it.

Step 4: Use more obstacles for the student to maneuver around while retrieving the object.

Step 5: Repeat Steps 2 through 4 except, after the student looks at the space between himself and the object, have the student close his eyes, then move to pick up the object with his eyes closed. Note: Be sure there is no peeking, and that the student estimates the space without counting steps. Also, don't use objects that can hurt the student if stepped on.

GUESSING TIME

Material:

- Wristwatch

Procedure:

Step 1: Throughout the day, ask the student to guess what time it is without looking at his watch.

Step 2: Begin with guessing the hour, then hour and minutes.

Step 3: Once the student guesses the time, have him locate the position of the sun (without looking directly at the sun), then at the watch to see how close he was to his estimate.

GETTING READY

Material:

- Clock

Procedure

Step 1: Have the student write down each activity needed to get ready before school.

Step 2: Have the student estimate how long each activity will take.

Step 3: Time each activity of the process to see how close the student's estimate is.

Step 4: Have the student decide how much more time or less time is needed to complete the different activities to getting ready.

Step 5: Have the student lengthen all activities to take more time. Have him estimate how much more time it will take.

Step 6: Have the student shorten all activities to take less time. Have him estimate how much less time it will take.

Step 7: Have the student mix up the times of the different parts. Make some shorter and some longer.

Note: Practice this activity on weekends or after school, not in the morning before school.

Always Late Lucy

The family expected her to always be late even when she wasn't. Getting ready in the morning always ended in an argument about how she made everyone else late. Everything her parents tried just created more frustration. She took the lateness with her when she became an adult and it has created much anxiety for her. One day she decided to try the strategies in this chapter and she was better able to manage her tardiness. She now is on time more often and she feels better about herself.

TROUBLESHOOTING

A student who has extreme difficulty with timing is usually identified long before he begins school. This is the child who is the last to wake up in the morning, and the last to get ready when the family is going somewhere. This child can become distracted easily when getting ready, and may find himself lost in thought without realizing the clock is ticking away. He loses all track of time.

Most of my good friends and family members who are frequently late have similar characteristics. Some of these characteristics are:

- Very high intelligence

- Musically gifted

- Very giving, and always wanting to help out

- Time is not a priority

- Would rather stop and chat than worry about the clock

- Get nervous or anxious when they must not be late

Some students pick up timing easily, and others work on it for a lifetime. Some students know exactly how many minutes they will be late. Some students have no idea that they are going to be late.

For students who have extreme difficulty with either arriving too early or too late, the strategies and techniques in this chapter will improve their ability to estimate time. The longer and more complicated the task, the more difficult time estimation will be.

STUDENTS WHO HAVE LITTLE TO NO IDEA OF WHEN THEY WILL BE LATE CAN HAVE BIG PROBLEMS IN LIFE.

Students who have no idea whether or not they will be late can have big problems later in life. Someday when they are on their own they will need to get to an appointment or to their jobs on time. In the future they may have a supervisor that emphasizes timeliness, and the boss may become critical of the students for things other than tardiness. Only extreme consequences for being late will have an effect on their internal clocks. These students need strategies to help them arrive at the correct times. Some ideas are:

- Have more than one alarm clock, placed away from the bed

- Estimate and be exact on how long each part of getting ready in the morning takes

- Do not go on social media or check email before you leave for an appointment

- Do not do any unplanned tasks when getting ready

- Do as many things as you can the day before to reduce the time it takes to get ready

SUMMARY

When students identify their priorities and then turn them into goals, they develop time management skills that will last a lifetime. The ideas in this chapter will be of value when doing homework, and they will aid the student in finding time to develop special talents. It is a wonderful gift you will have given your student, allowing him to excel beyond his expectations.

REVIEW

Visual Skills

- Binocularity

- Accommodation

- Temporal Localization
- Temporal Organization
- Temporal Orientation

Time

- 10 to 15 minutes daily on timing techniques
- Daily use of timing components

Coaching

- Use time in daily conversation
- Use positive coaching to help students discover how to understand time

Components

- Wrist Watch
- Bedside Alarm Clock
- Stopwatch
- Digital Devices

Building Skills

- Take advantage of the spare moments given in class
- Be sure the study hall is productive and is not a social hour

Practice

- Time Estimation
- Space Estimation
- Guessing Time
- Getting Ready

Troubleshooting

- For students who cannot grasp or estimate time well, develop strategies for reminders about time

10

STAYING ORGANIZED

CREATE FOCUSED PRODUCTIVITY

Organization isn't about perfection. It's about efficiency, reducing stress and clutter, saving time and money and improving your overall quality of life.

— Christina Scalise

Students can surpass their expectations for learning ability by building a schedule. This organizational skill results in productive quality time for both work and play. The Visual Secrets presented in this book will guide coaches to help students achieve this. The techniques discussed in Chapters 4 through 8 are used to improve a student's academic performance and build self-confidence in his ability to excel. It may be overwhelming to figure out how to accomplish these activities. Highlighted in this chapter is a proven system for helping both students and their coaches be more productive. For over 30 years my patients have achieved improved school performance, less homework, and better grades. I have had the pleasure of seeing them go on to become successful adults.

Ralph Waldo Emerson said, "A good system shortens the road to the goal." The following is a system that students can use to be better organized, so they can complete homework quicker and have more quality time.

With good organization skills your student will have more productive time to do the things he wants to do. This will help him have a more positive attitude when some assignments or Visual Secrets activities are difficult. To build self-esteem, point out situations where using Visual Secrets has made an assignment or activity easier or take less time. His new skills will give him time to develop his areas of interest. He will begin achieving. This, in turn, will have a snowball effect on his self-confidence. Both his coach and he will see that he can surpass expectations and be successful at whatever he chooses to do.

> WITH GOOD ORGANIZATION SKILLS YOUR STUDENT WILL HAVE MORE PRODUCTIVE TIME TO DO THE THINGS HE WANTS TO DO. THIS WILL HELP HIM HAVE A MORE POSITIVE ATTITUDE WHEN SOME ASSIGNMENTS OR VISUAL SECRETS ACTIVITIES ARE DIFFICULT.

VISUAL SKILLS FOR ORGANIZATION:

Visual Skill	Definition
Saccades	The ability to shift the eye fixation from one object to another
Binocularity	The ability to use the two eyes together so they send the same message to the brain at the same time
Accommodation	The ability to keep an image in focus when viewed up close
Visual Association	Relating one object or idea to another
Visual Categorization	Grouping similar items or ideas together

Visualization	The ability to see pictures of objects with the eyes closed
Visual Memory	Being able to recall previously viewed information or scenes
Spatial Organization	The ability to arrange information
Allocentric Localization	How objects in the surrounding area relate to each other
Visual Identification, Matching and Discrimination of Size, Shape, and Space	Knowing similarities and differences of what is being thought of or looked at
Visual Figure Ground	Being aware of a viewed object without letting the background interfere

Saccades: Allows for quick assessment of the task.

Binocularity: Helps judge where things are.

Accommodation: Keeps the whole task in focus.

Visual Association: Allows the student to relate similar tasks.

Visual Categorization: Allows for grouping of similar tasks.

Visualization: Gives the student the ability to see the "big picture" of what needs to be accomplished.

Visual Memory: Helps in remembering where everything is that the task requires.

Spatial Organization: Aids in understanding what fits where.

Allocentric Localization: Gives information on how different objects relate to each other spatially.

Visual Identification, Matching and Discrimination of Size, Shape, and Space: The ability to notice what goes together and what does not. This is beneficial when organizing an area.

Visual Figure Ground: The ability to see the entire task that needs to be accomplished, and determining the best place to start.

TIME

When building good learning skills, work on the activities for about 20 minutes, then take a physical break. You will get further with small steps than by trying to do all of it at once. Some activities can be turned into a weekly family game night. Use 30 minutes a day to practice organizing something, such as the backpack, a drawer, the homework folder, etc.

COACHING

When helping guide the student to use the Visual Secret techniques in Chapters 4 through 8, do not have other siblings present. Sibling competition can be negative, especially when the student who needs the help has a more difficult time with the activities.

When the student begins an organizing task, ask him how he would break it down to complete it instead of telling him how it should be done.

Alex's room was constantly cluttered.

Every space that was designated as Alex's space was a mess. He could never find anything. Everything had dust on it. He threw all of his clothes on the floor and had no idea which ones were clean or dirty. He never made his bed. When he went to college his mother wouldn't even go into his dorm room because it was so awful. Everyone commented on the mess he lived in. One day he decided to change and began using better organizing strategies and slowly began to take care of his space. This had a huge positive impact on his attitude and he was less depressed. He stopped misplacing things. He learned that life is easier when things are organized.

COMPONENTS

BREAKING DOWN TASKS

To develop the needed skills for learning, pick one subject at a time. Don't try to do them all at once. Pick the easiest subject for your student first, then the second-easiest, and so on. Sometimes it is best to work on the activities during summer break, when things are less hectic. Do them in the morning when your student is rested. See Appendix #6 for how to break down and complete the activities in Chapters 4 through 8.

KEEPING TRACK OF EVERYTHING

- Do you have homework?
- What is your homework assignment?
- Where is your homework?
- Did you turn in your homework?

These are not uncommon questions from the parent when it is time to do homework. Let's first determine how to keep track of the assignments, which can be quite challenging and frustrating for students, parents, and teachers. When my kids were going through school, the school administration decided that the best way for the students to be organized was for them to use a daily planner. Every student was given a daily planner and was required to use it. With this planner, the responsibility to know and complete assignments fell on the student. This left everyone else "off the hook," so to speak. Andrew decided he could just keep everything in his head which worked most of the time. Clarice was good at remembering to put all of her assignments in her planner. Natalie's high-level of attention to detail also made it easy for her to use a daily planner.

People organize their thoughts and learn tasks in different ways. With this in mind, it is critical to determine what will work for your specific student. Personally, I like to look at calendars one month at a time. Our family kept a monthly "dry erase" calendar on the refrigerator, and we color-coded it for each person's activities. Thinking ahead makes it easier to plan for the due date. Assignments can be started earlier and accomplished a little at a time when there is a free moment. This helps avoid the last-minute crisis and being caught with too little time to get them finished. Others may prefer daily or weekly planners. Figure out what works for your individual student.

A wide variety of calendar applications for digital devices are available that provide different ways to keep track of assignments. Some will give you daily reminders and help break down the big assignments into smaller chunks. This helps reduce the feeling of being overwhelmed, which can stifle the process of getting things finished on time. If your student's system doesn't work, find a different one.

ACCOUNTABILITY REMINDERS

What happens if your student doesn't write down the assignment in the organizer? This is where accountability comes in. The teacher must be part of the team. Before the school day finishes, ask the teacher to sign his initials on the assignment book to ensure the assignments are in the planner. When the student gets home and the planner has been initialed, he gets a reward for remembering to have the teacher check the correctly recorded assignment. Some kids cannot remember, so ask the teacher to help prompt your student. With daily checks, the student will learn the pattern and begin recording his assignments consistently.

TURNING IN HOMEWORK

Finding the assignments to be completed and turning them in can sometimes be an issue for students. In these cases, the student should help decide the best place to keep assignments.

One suggestion is a homework folder. Make it a good-quality, fun-looking one that cannot get missed or mixed up with others. Maybe have a note on it—*DON'T FORGET ME!* Some planners have sleeves so both completed homework and incomplete homework can all be in one place. Another possibility is having a special place in the backpack.

With assignments, follow-up and accountability are important in order to create a pattern. Assistance from the teacher may be needed to check that all of the assignments are in the folder at the end of the day. The parent will need to check to see if the completed assignments are in the folder before bedtime. Students will even need to double-check the folder in the morning. Give a reward if all completed assignments are in the right place, and give a consequence if they are not.

FREE TIME

Once homework is getting done in a shorter time, the student will begin to build confidence and have more free time. When this happens, sit down with your student to help him develop goals for what to do with that spare time. Maybe he wants to improve an athletic ability, or has developed an interest for reading and wants to read more, or would like to spend more time with friends. All of these are great goals to further solidify new self-confidence. Following through with these goals also establishes a good work ethic. Working hard for short periods of time should be rewarded with a positive activity. Make a list of positive rewards that your student will enjoy.

SPARE MOMENTS COUNT

Besides tracking assignments, encourage your student to take advantage of spare moments in the classroom when others may still be finishing an in-class assignment. Have students create a system so they can take out a homework assignment to work on during spare moments. Have him do shorter assignments first. This does two things. It helps create a sense of accomplishment and it reduces the number of books to be brought home.

COMPLETING EXTRA-CREDIT ASSIGNMENTS CAN BUILD SELF-CONFIDENCE, IMPROVE THE TEACHER'S ATTITUDE TOWARD THE STUDENT, AND RAISE HIS GRADE.

Sometimes teachers offer extra-credit activities. If regular assignments are complete, suggest to your student to consider attempting some of the extra-credit ones. Have him do one in an area that he enjoys. Completing extra-credit assignments can build self-confidence, improve the teacher's attitude toward the student, and raise his grade.

BUILDING ORGANIZATIONAL SKILLS
ORGANIZING THE STUDENT'S ROOM

Materials:

- The Student's Space

Procedure:

Step 1: The student is to give all of the areas within his space an organization grade. At a minimum the following should be on the list:

- Bed

- Dresser

- Closet

- Study area

Step 2: Have the student reorganize the space that had the best grade.

Step 3: Discuss the changed organization with the student. Have him decide if he thinks it is improved. Repeat with the next-best-graded spaces until all of the spaces are reorganized.

ATTRIBUTE BLOCKS

This technique was discussed in detail in Chapter 7. It trains the concept of categorization and association.

PARQUETRY BLOCKS

This technique was discussed in detail in Chapter 7. It trains the concept of categorization and association. Emphasize the identification, matching, and determination of the space between the blocks. Vary the spaces between the blocks and encourage the student to match both the blocks and their exact positions.

WHAT'S WRONG?

Materials:

- A "What's Wrong with the Picture" Game (for examples, search online for "what's wrong with this picture")

Procedure:

Step 1: Play the game.
Step 2: Recreate the game using a room in the house.
Step 3: Place 3 items in the wrong spot.
Step 4: See if the student can figure out which items are in the wrong spot.
Step 5: Increase the number of items used.

PRACTICE

BACK PACK

Materials:

- Backpack

- Items in backpack

Procedure:

Step 1: Time can be a factor when the student cannot get organized. Try to find 30 minutes in the evening that allow for the student to reorganize his backpack and homework folder. At first, have the student remove all items and ask him to determine how to replace them in an organized way. Use positive coaching with probing questions.

Step 2: Repeat until organizing the backpack takes less than 5 minutes and does not require any coaching.

PLANNER

Materials:

- Planner

- Markers

- Fun writing pen

Procedure:

Step 1: Have the student decide which planner style works the best: daily, weekly, or monthly.

Step 2: Have the student make a list of all that goes into the planner.

Step 3: Put the list into categories.

Step 4: Have the student decide which color to highlight the different categories. Examples of categories are: assignments, sport practice, fun time, special events.

Step 5: At the end of each school day, ask the teacher to initial each day that the assignments are correctly listed in the planner.

Step 6: Daily, the coach initials that the planner is correct and up-to-date for all categories.

Step 7: When the assignments are always correctly recorded for 90 days, then only initial them weekly, then monthly, then quarterly.

HOMEWORK FOLDER

Materials:

- Homework folder

Procedure:

Step 1: Have the student choose a folder he likes. Encourage him to be sure it has one space for completed homework and one space for homework that needs to be done.

Step 2: Prepare the student to know how to match and record the finished and unfinished homework with the planner.

Step 3: Have the student record in the planner (with a check mark) each time he reviews the homework folder. Be sure it is reviewed at least three times daily. In the morning, just before school ends, and just before bedtime are recommended times.

Step 4: Reward the student daily for three checkmarks on the previous day. Give extra rewards for more than three checkmarks.

SCHOOL LOCKER AND DESK

Materials:

- Student's desk

- School locker

- Locker organizers

Procedure:

Step 1: Schedule a time with the student to reorganize his locker and/or desk. Record these times in the student's planner so he knows when to expect it. Do this at the beginning and middle of each quarter. Let the student do the organizing. Coaches, don't touch anything...let the student do it all. Be a positive coach by asking probing questions. Don't tell him what to do with the items in the locker and/or desk.

Step 2: Take a picture of the finished product.

Step 3: Enlarge the picture and place it on the mirror of the bathroom in which the student gets ready.

Step 4: Once a week, ask the student how close the picture is to the organized desk and/or locker.

Step 5: Give a reward for the locker and/or desk matching the organized picture at the quarterly review.

CLASS NOTES AND BOOKS

Materials:

- Class notes

- Class books

- Class folders

- Class binders

Procedure:

Step 1: Have the student choose folders and binders he will use for each class.

Step 2: Have the student make a list of any book, folder, workbook, or binder that will be used for each class.

Step 3: Keep the list with the planner.

Step 4: If the student can easily keep these items where he has decided they belong, have him check his list weekly. If not, it needs to be done daily until they are all in the right place at all times.

TROUBLESHOOTING

When the task to organize is too overwhelming, the student feels defeated even before beginning. This creates a situation of avoidance. The book *The Life-Changing Magic of Tidying Up: The Japanese Art of Decluttering and Organizing* by Marie Kondo explains how to accomplish big tasks when it seems impossible.[41] She recommends organizing similar items at the same time. For example, do all of your clothes at one time. She does not recommend going drawer by drawer.

> WHEN THE TASK TO ORGANIZE IS TOO OVERWHELMING, THE STUDENT FEELS DEFEATED EVEN BEFORE BEGINNING. THIS CREATES A SITUATION OF AVOIDANCE.

In Chapter 14 of her book *See It, Say It, Do It!* Dr. Lynn Hellerstein describes how to visualize the tasks to be done.[42] She suggests breaking down the tasks into small parts, and taking the least important tasks off the to-do list by visualizing them being thrown out a window. This helps to remove the student's mind clutter so he can focus on the important tasks.

SUMMARY

To help your student surpass expectations, guide him to be better organized. Do this by knowing which systems work best for him. Get help from teachers when necessary. Coach him about using spare time wisely, both at home and in the classroom. Help him realize success and reach goals, which will in turn give him confidence to be successful in what he chooses.

Once students learn the Visual Secrets in Chapters 4 through 8, they will have less homework and more free time. To begin guiding your student through these activities, work on one area at a time. Have the student choose the subject he wants to improve upon and begin with that one. It may surprise the coach, but most students usually pick their best subject first. The coach might prefer the student start with his worst subject. However, starting with the student's best subject is fine because the success realized with an easy subject will keep him positive when working on more difficult ones.

REVIEW

Visual Skills

- Saccades
- Binocularity
- Accommodation
- Association
- Categorization
- Visualization
- Visual Memory
- Spatial Organization
- Allocentric Localization

Time

- 20 minutes daily to practice Visual Secret Techniques
- 30 minutes daily to organize one thing

Coaching

- Do the Visual Secret Techniques with a positive approach
- Do not do the techniques with other siblings; keep them one-on-one

Components

- Breaking Down Tasks
- Keeping Track of Everything
- Accountability Reminders
- Turning In Homework
- Free Time
- Spare Moments Count

Building Skills

- Organizing the Student's Room
- Attribute Blocks
- Parquetry Blocks
- What's Wrong?

Practice

- Backpack

- Planner

- Homework folder

- School locker and desk

- Class notes and books

Troubleshooting

- *The Life-Changing Magic of Tidying Up: The Japanese Art of Decluttering and Organizing* by Marie Kondo

- *See It. Say It. Do It!* By Lynn Hellerstein

11

WORKING SMARTER, NOT HARDER

CHOOSE YOUR LIFE

I manage my time by prioritizing tasks,
working smarter not harder, and by
avoiding procrastination.

— Jeet Banerjee

Visual Secrets for School Success is about working smarter, not harder. The techniques help students use visual skills at maximum capacity to be more efficient and effective when completing assignments. This allows students to surpass not only their parents' and teachers' expectations, but also their own. Efficiency with high-level performance has a positive impact on a student's self-confidence. This chapter will give techniques to help build self-confidence for students when working on the Visual Secret activities and for everyday living.

VISUAL SKILLS FOR KNOWING ONE'S SELF:

Visual Skill	Definition
Eye Movements	The ability to hold fixation on what is looked at, to follow moving targets, and shift the eye fixation from one object to another
Accommodation	The ability to keep an image in focus when viewed up close
Binocularity	The ability to use the two eyes together so they send the same message to the brain at the same time
Spatial and Temporal Orientation	The synchrony between the eye-brain process and the environment for maintaining self-position and the internal clock system
Spatial and Temporal Organization	The eye-brain process of comparing events as they relate to when they happen
Visualization	The ability to see pictures with the eyes closed
Visual Memory	The ability to recall a viewed image over an extended period of time
Egocentric Localization	Knowing where your center is

Eye Movements: Taking in the situation, seeing what is, and seeing what can be begins with being able to see "the big picture." When the eyes move inefficiently, it is difficult to process the entire environment to make accurate judgments and decisions.

Accommodation: Being able to stay focused long enough to figure out what needs to be accomplished is important to help students set the stage for successfully completing tasks.

Binocularity: Depth perception reduces the amount of visual stress. This supports better orientation and organization of self.

Spatial and Temporal Orientation: Knowing how much is involved and how long it will take to complete a task develops the student's ability to make decisions and to plan what he can and cannot do.

Spatial and Temporal Organization: This is judging how space and time are organized. Being skilled in this area helps with judgments in many areas. Completing tasks in a timely manner can be more difficult when there is more stress.

> UNDERSTANDING WHERE AND WHO YOU ARE IS CRITICAL IN ORDER TO RELATE THIS UNDERSTANDING TO OTHERS AND IN VARIOUS SITUATIONS.

Visualization: Seeing one's self in a positive way improves self-confidence.

Visual Memory: This skill helps when remembering fun events and positive situations.

Egocentric Localization: Understanding where and who you are is critical in order to relate this understanding to others and in various situations.

TIME

Spend about 20 minutes a day working on the *Visual Secrets for School Success*. Each day find five positive things the student is doing well. Spend time noting it in detail, and leave one quote per day for the student to discover.

COACHING

Self Confidence Rules for the Coach

1. Ask, don't tell, the student to perform a task. (Suggestion: Ask a question about the task you want the student to perform. Ask, "Is the dog dish empty?" instead of saying, "Feed the dog." Ask, "How is your homework coming along?" instead of saying, "Do your homework.")

2. Try to point out what is right about the student's performance, not what is wrong. (Example: "You got six of the seven letters correct when spelling *reptile*," vs. "You spelled *reptile* wrong.")

3. Help the student discover how to solve his problem by listening to him talk about it. Then ask what he thinks should be done about the problem. Don't give suggestions on how to fix the problem; let him make suggestions.

4. Do not label your student as "the smart one," or "the artist," or any other label. It fixes his mindset and stifles his ability to work hard to achieve any task presented.[43]

5. Do not compare your student to other students, especially his friends or siblings.

6. Do not criticize the student or call him or her a name, such as, "You are not that smart," or, "You are not good at math," or, "You are lazy."

7. Do not say the student is a "good" or "bad" student. This label creates a perceived expectation that they feel they need to live up to.[43]

8. When talking about a completed project, use a lot of details and talk about the effort the student put into the activity. Often remark how hard he is working on the assignment.

COMPONENTS

ATTRIBUTES

Make a list of the student's positive attributes or strengths. Make the list lengthy. Personality traits, specific abilities in sports, skills with hobbies, or appreciation of nature or animals are areas that can be considered.

ATTITUDE

Both the coach and the student need to have positive attitudes when doing fun activities and when working on difficult ones. Negative thinking is like a big wall. It shuts you down. It stops you from accomplishing goals, and blocks your ability to move forward to accomplish life goals. This is true for learning, relationships, and finding happiness. Negative attitudes hurt the student's ability to reach his full potential. Come up with a way to remind each other when the attitude is negative. Create ways to change the attitude. Some ideas are as follows:

- Take a mini break and talk about each other's attributes.

- Make the learning space more fun. Use ideas in Chapter 2.

- Use quotes to inspire students.

- Visualize or imagine a scene that has been a positive experience.

- Don't allow negative words.

- Define negative versus positive thoughts.

- Coaches, be the student's biggest fan.

- Reward positive behavior rather than punishing negative actions.

- Take out the student's baby picture album and talk about how happy you were when they arrived. Discuss cute things they did as a baby.

> **Denise was depressed.**
>
> Denise felt bad about herself. She struggled in school. Her parents were frustrated with the daily challenges of completing homework. She did not take pride in her appearance. She had difficulty making friends. She seemed to have a bad attitude about everything. One day her parents began to change how they spoke to Denise, and she began to change. With encouraging parents, she felt better about herself. She put more effort into school and her self-appearance. She began to make friends, which was also a positive influence. Slowly she began to succeed and then improve her grades. Her class voted her most likely to succeed, and she went on to college.

BUILDING SKILLS

MOTIVATION

Help motivate your student in subjects that may be more difficult than others by using positive quotes and sayings. Relate that particular skill to different daily living activities. Pick up a hobby that helps develop that skill. Guide your student to create a positive attitude toward the specific subject. The "feel-good" button is a huge plus when trying to overcome a difficult task. Once overcoming a hard task, emphasis should be put on how hard the student worked and point out what was accomplished by that hard work. When things get easier, continue to illustrate how the hard work paid off by saying, "Do you remember when things like this were more difficult than they are now? It's because you worked hard and now you are reaping the benefits."

PRIORITIES

To motivate a student to value organization and time, begin by determining his priorities. What is important to him? What does he want to improve in his life? What makes him happy, and what makes him sad? Talk about what happens when he has more time versus less time. What are his hobbies and sport activities? Does he want to be able to spend more time with family and friends? Ask the student to describe what a perfect day would be like. Have him visualize himself doing something fun. Visualizing was discussed in Chapter 5.

GOALS

Once the student's priorities are defined and verbalized, have him write them down as goals. Put the priorities and goals in order of most importance to him. An example of a priority might be, "My parents are the most important people in my life." A goal related to this priority might be, "I would like to spend more quality time with my parents." (Yes, the teen student may exchange "friends" for parents.)

To create a positive attitude about valuing time, place written quotations in the student's bedroom and bathroom. As he begins his day, he will see them while he is getting ready. Also put them in his homework assignment folder, backpack, lunch bag, and locker. Below are some motivating quotes that may inspire your student to value his time. Include some motivational sayings to help him feel good about the effort he is making to improve himself, to save time, and to make life easier.

PRACTICE

POSITIVE THINKING

Take every opportunity to build motivation and self-esteem in your student.

QUOTES

Leave quotes in special places. The following are some ideas depending on the area your student has difficulty with.

- Time

  - ○ "Every second is of infinite value." Jonathan Wolfgang von Goethe

- Inspiration

  - ○ "Let your smile change the world but don't let the world change your smile." Connor Franta

- Trying Hard

  - ○ "Anyone who has never made a mistake, has never tried anything new." Albert Einstein

- Success

  - ○ "If you can dream it, you can do it." Walt Disney

  - ○ "The only time you find success before work is in the dictionary." May V. Smith

  - ○ "Successful people do what unsuccessful people are not willing to do." Jim Rohn

  - ○ "Success seems to be connected with action. Successful people keep moving. They make mistakes, but they don't quit." Conrad Hilton

  - ○ "If you really want to do something, you'll find a way. If you don't, you'll find an excuse." Jim Rohn

- Spelling

  - ○ "Spell well, or be thought of as less intelligent than you actually are." Brenda Montecalvo

- o "When our spelling is perfect, it's invisible. But when it's flawed, it prompts strong negative associations." Marilyn vos Savant

- o "Be mindful of your spelling…auto correct is not always write." Jesse Neo

- Writing

  - o "Writing is easy. All you have to do is cross out the wrong words." Mark Twain

  - o "The hardest part of writing is just before you begin." Anonymous

  - o "Start writing, no matter what. The water does not flow until the faucet is turned on." Louis L'Amour

  - o "Writing is thinking on paper." William Zinsser

  - o "You might not write well every day, but you can always edit a bad page. You can't edit a blank page." Jodi Picoult

- Math

  - o "Math and science are the lifeblood of the future." Bob Becker

  - o "Give me a lever long enough and a fulcrum on which to place it, and I shall move the world." Archimedes

  - o "The essence of mathematics is not to make simple things complicated, but to make complicated things simple." Stan Gudder

  - o "Think of a number. Double it. Add six, then half it. Subtract the number you started with. Your number is three." Anonymous

  - o "Math is like ice cream, with more flavors than you can imagine—and if all you ever do is textbook math, that's like eating broccoli-flavored ice cream." Denise Gaskins

- Reading

  o "Today a reader, tomorrow a leader." Margaret Fuller

  o "Once you learn to read, you will be forever free." Frederick Douglas

  o "Reading is essential for those who seek to rise above the ordinary." Jim Rohn

  o "If you don't like to read, you haven't found the right book." J.K. Rowling

  o "Reading is a discount ticket to everywhere." Mary Schmich

VISUAL SECRETS

The activities on handwriting in Chapter 4 showed students how to have more legible penmanship. With this skill, writing assignments will be completed faster and with ease. A student's thoughts can dwell on composition topics and structure instead of focusing on the discomfort and difficulty of handwriting. The student will be proud of his improved handwriting.

The activities on spelling in Chapter 5 showed how students can become good spellers, and that it does not take a long time to learn to spell words correctly. Getting A's on spelling tests will give students higher self-confidence at an early age. Good spellers spend less time looking up words, which will result in better grades on writing assignments. Being a good speller gives a better first impression, and builds self-confidence that will last a lifetime. One day maybe your student will surpass everyone's expectations and win the national spelling bee.

Composition is a skill few students develop well. Use the ideas in Chapter 6 to become a great writer. When the time comes to complete a college application or an essay for a scholarship, the student with well-developed composition skills will have a higher chance of success. Scholarships are often awarded based on essays that are submitted to a review committee, and learning to write an interesting essay is an important skill. Can students learn this? Yes, they can, and it makes them feel proud to be recognized for a scholastic achievement. Having the ability to write excellent compositions gives students an extra edge as they start college. Better writers have more self-confidence and feel better about themselves. These students have more opportunities in life because of their excellent composition skills. One day, they may become famous authors. Anything is possible. We are only limited by our imagination of what can be.

Who wants to be the last person to finish a timed math test? For the student who finishes last, this can decrease his self-confidence, and he quickly learns to dislike math. When a student loathes the idea of completing a math assignment, the poor attitude toward the subject interferes with the ability to learn math concepts. The math ideas in Chapter 7 show how to complete math facts quickly. The suggested games give the student better visual skills to judge space accurately and learn to assess and measure that space with ease. Today we have machines telling us the answers to math problems. When a 10 percent discount should be given on a store purchase, often the cashier cannot calculate the discount if the cash register doesn't display it. What about tipping at a restaurant? How many people need to use a calculator to determine the amount of the tip? When having dinner in a group, the person who calculates the 18% tip in his or her head is perceived as smarter. Many higher paying jobs require good math skills and the understanding of math concepts. Using the ideas in the math chapter will help the student achieve a better life by giving him more options. He doesn't have to settle for a job he doesn't like just to get by. He can achieve the career of his dreams and be happy doing it.

> READING IS THE MOST IMPORTANT ACADEMIC SKILL IN WHICH TO EXCEL BECAUSE NEARLY EVERYTHING ONE DOES TO GET AHEAD IN LIFE REQUIRES THE ABILITY TO READ AND COMPREHEND.

Reading is the most important academic skill in which to excel because nearly everything one does to get ahead in life requires the ability to read and comprehend. This is more difficult for a poor reader. Enjoyment of reading gives the student a lifetime skill that helps him entertain himself without depending on a digital device, and it allows him to be a lifetime learner. It makes him feel good about himself and his ability, and it can take him anywhere he wants to go in his mind's eye. If he doesn't know an answer to a question, he can read something to figure it out by himself. Being a good reader leads to more possibilities, better jobs, more enjoyment in learning, and a better life. Completing the reading activities in Chapter 8 will help your student surpass his expectations.

TROUBLESHOOTING

Some students who have had years of struggling to succeed are not very motivated to keep trying. Who could blame them when all attempts to complete assignments are returned with red marks and parents berating them for not trying hard enough? Teachers are frustrated with them because all efforts to teach them have not worked. Slowly, these situations wear down a student's motivation to try, and they don't feel good about themselves.

These students want to be successful. They need a positive coach, and they need someone to believe in their ability to do well.

Find out what your student likes, or what interests him. Make time to build skills in this area in a way that is fun and interesting to the student. With lots of encouragement from the coach, he will find a foothold on the first rung of the ladder leading out of a defeating environment, and begin to do well in an area in which he is interested.

SUMMARY

With high-level visual skills that students can use for all areas of academic requirements, they will achieve success in school. That success will lead to wonderful opportunities after formal school is completed. Students will be rewarded with respect, promotions, and a satisfying lifestyle. Knowing the Visual Secrets in this book will lead to a better life. Enjoy your future of learning!

REVIEW

Visual Skills

- Eye Movements
- Accommodation
- Spatial and Temporal Orientation
- Spatial and Temporal Organization
- Egocentric Localization

Time

- 20 minutes per day for Visual Secrets
- Five positive statements per day about what the student does well
- One quote per day for the student to discover

Coaching

- Ask questions
- Show what's right
- Encourage self-discovery
- No labels
- Don't compare
- No criticism
- No name-calling
- Detailed admiration

Components

- Attributes
- Attitudes

Building Skills

- Motivation
- Priorities
- Goals

Practice

- Positive Thinking
- Quotes for Motivation
- Visual Secret Skills
  - Handwriting
  - Spelling
  - Composition

- ○ Math
- ○ Reading

Troubleshooting

- Discover an interest and find time to develop it
- Encourage the effort to learn a new skill

APPENDICES

APPENDIX #1
OPTOMETRISTS WHO CHECK
FOR VISUAL SKILLS

The following are groups of optometrists who check for visual skills needed for learning:

- College of Optometrists in Vision Development: https://www.covd.org

- Optometric Extension Program: www.oepf.org

- College of Syntonic Optometry: https://csovision.org

- Neuro-Optometric Rehabilitation Association: https://noravisionrehab.org

- Vision Leads Foundation: www.visionleadsfoundation.com

- www.vision3d.com

- Facebook page "Vision Therapy Parents Unite"

- Facebook page "VTODs on Facebook"

APPENDIX #2
VISUAL SKILLS

- Visual Motor
  - Eye Movements
    - Fixation
    - Pursuits
    - Saccades
  - Accommodation
    - Flexibility
  - Convergence and Divergence
    - Amplitude
    - Posture
    - Flexibility
- Visual Sensory
  - Acuity
    - Far
    - Intermediate
    - Near

- Accommodation
  - Amplitude
  - Posture
- Fusion
  - First Degree
  - Second Degree
  - Third Degree (Stereopsis)
- Visual Fields
  - Central
  - Peripheral
  - Blind spot
- Visual Thinking
  - Sensory Integration
    - Orientation
    - Organization
    - Reaction time
    - Peripheral/Central Organization
  - Perceptual Skills
    - Laterality
    - Directionality
    - Visualization
  - Cognitive Skills
    - Visual Memory
    - Categorization

- Association
- Figure Ground
- Visual Closure
- Identification
  - Size
  - Shape
  - Space
- Matching
  - Size
  - Shape
  - Space
- Discrimination
  - Size
  - Shape
  - Space

APPENDIX #3
QUESTIONS TO ASK THE
EYE DOCTOR

All eye doctors check for 20/20 eyesight and eye health problems during routine examinations. However, not all eye doctors measure the visual skills of tracking, focusing, eye teaming (3-D) and visual perception. All of these visual skills are important for optimal learning. Up to 80% of children with some type of learning problem have visual skills that are below normal, even though they may have 20/20 eyesight and healthy eyes. Your eye doctor should be able to determine if your child has problems with any of the visual skills important for learning, or should refer you to another eye doctor for those assessments. There are several evidence-based age normative tests that accurately measure the levels of visual skills a child should have achieved.

A comprehensive eye health and visual evaluation should take from 30 minutes to one hour to complete. If a problem is identified, additional testing can take up to two hours.

Ask your eye doctor the following questions to ensure you are receiving the very best eye health and vision evaluation for your child:

1. Will you do any visual perceptual testing during the eye examination?

2. Do you measure for tracking, focusing, and eye teaming (3-D) problems?

3. Do you feel that vision problems, other than reduced 20/20 eyesight, can affect school performance?

4. Do you provide in-office optometric vision therapy?

5. Does your office refer to an optometrist that provides optometric vision therapy when you find a vision problem that can affect learning?

6. Are the tests for tracking, focusing, eye teaming, and visual perception done before the eyes are dilated?

7. Will the time with the eye doctor take longer than 15 minutes?

8. Is the eye doctor certified in any area of vision development or visual rehabilitation?

9. Do you check the eyes at near before putting drops in the eyes?

A "No" response to any of the above questions may indicate that all of the visual skills for optimal performance and good learning might not be evaluated during the eye health and vision examination. An eye doctor that provides these extra tests, or refers to doctors that do, is committed to ensuring patients receive a complete visual skill evaluation. The eye doctor that does more in-depth testing for these problems is often a Fellow of the College of Optometrists in Vision Development (FCOVD), which means the doctor is board certified in the area of vision therapy. For a list of board-certified eye doctors in your area go to www.covd.org. Other good resources about vision and learning are www.thevisiontherapycenter.com and Facebook page "Vision Therapy Parents Unite".

APPENDIX #4
COMPONENTS OF A
COMPREHENSIVE EYE
EXAMINATION

A comprehensive eye health and vision examination consists of many tests, such as the following:

Eye Health

- Dilated fundus examination of inner part of the eye, including the lens and retina
- Complete health examination of the outer part of the eye, including lids, lashes and cornea
- A visual field screening on each eye. If there are headaches or history of brain injury, then a full threshold visual field should be completed for patients over age 6.

Visual Sensory

- Visual acuity at distance (6 meters) and near (40 centimeters)
- Fusion assessment by a cover test at distance and at near

Visual Motor

- Fixations, pursuits and saccades (at near)
  - Each eye alone
  - Both eyes together
- Accommodation of each eye
- Binocularity, by either stereoscopic or phoropter testing

Visual Thinking

- Visual Motor Integration (VMI) Test
- Test of Visual-Perceptual Skills (TVPS)
- Piaget Left/Right Awareness Test
- Wold Sentence Copy Test

Note: This is a partial list, and there can be additions and substitutions to the list. This list includes the minimum tests required to determine visual skill performance.

APPENDIX #5
ACTIVITY RESOURCES

- Slanted work surface - visit Visual Edge® Slant Board (www.visualedgesb.com)

- Geoboard – visit Walmart (www.walmart.com)

- Attribute Blocks - visit EAI Education (www.eaieducation.com)

- Parquetry Blocks – visit Christianbook (www.christianbook.com)

APPENDIX #6
12-WEEK VISUAL
SECRETS PROGRAM

Week 1	Time	Chapter	Spelling Activities
Day 1	2 hours	2	Setting up Study Space
Day 2	10 min.	5	Stacking Cups
Day 2	15 min.	5	MONTECALVO Spelling Technique for 10 words
Day 3-5	10 min.	5	Parquetry Block Memory
Day 3-5	15 min.	5	MONTECALVO Spelling Technique for 10 words
Day 6	20 min.	5	Practice Spelling Test
Day 7			Enjoy Family Time and Play Time

Week 2	Time	Chapter	Spelling Activities
Day 1-5	20 min.	5	MONTECALVO Spelling Technique for all words
Day 6	15 min.	5	Practice Spelling Test
Day 7			Enjoy Family Time and Play Time

Week 3	Time	Chapter	Spelling Activities
Day 1	15 min.	5	Commonly Misspelled words
Day 2-3	20 min.	5	MONTECALVO Spelling Technique for all words
Day 4	15 min.	5	Practice Spelling Test
Day 5	15 min.	5	Commonly Misspelled Words
Day 6	15 min.	5	Practice Spelling Test
Day 7			Enjoy Family Time and Play Time

Week 4	Time	Chapter	Math Activities
Day 1	15 min.	7	Counting Steps; Step 1-3
Day 1	15 min.	7	Measuring things
Day 2	15 min.	7	Counting Steps; Step 1-3
Day 2	15 min.	7	Dice Game
Day 3	15 min.	7	Counting Steps; Step 4
Day 3	15 min.	7	100 Squares
Day 4	15 min.	7	Counting Steps; Step 4
Day 4	15 min.	7	Puzzles
Day 5	15 min.	7	Counting Steps; Step 5
Day 5	15 min.	7	Perfect 10 Magic Trick
Day 6	15 min.	7	Counting Steps; Step 5
Day 6	15 min.	7	Dice Game
Day 7			Enjoy Family Time and Play Time

Week 5	Time	Chapter	Math Activities
Day 1	15 min.	7	Body Movement and Multiplication
Day 1	15 min.	7	Dr. M's Multiplication Math Facts Technique "2s"
Day 2	15 min.	7	Geometry Game
Day 2	15 min.	7	Dr. M's Multiplication Math Facts Technique "5s"
Day 3	15 min.	7	Body Movement and Multiplication
Day 3	15 min.	7	Dr. M's Multiplication Math Facts Technique "10s"
Day 4	15 min.	7	Geometry Game
Day 4	15 min.	7	Dr. M's Multiplication Math Facts Technique "3s"
Day 5	15 min.	7	Parquetry Blocks
Day 5	15 min.	7	Dr. M's Multiplication Math Facts Technique "4s"
Day 6	15 min.	7	Attribute Blocks
Day 6	15 min.	7	Dr. M's Multiplication Math Facts Technique "6s"
Day 7			Enjoy Family Time and Play Time

Week 6	Time	Chapter	Math Activities
Day 1	15 min.	7	Math Stars "2 – 4"
Day 1	15 min.	7	Dr. M's Multiplication Math Facts Technique "7s"
Day 2	15 min.	7	Math Stars "5 – 7"
Day 2	15 min.	7	Dr. M's Multiplication Math Facts Technique "8s"
Day 3	15 min.	7	Math Stars "8 – 9"
Day 3	15 min.	7	Dr. M's Multiplication Math Facts Technique "9s"
Day 4	15 min.	7	Math Stars "2-9"
Day 4	15 min.	7	Dr. M's Multiplication Math Facts Random "2s – 10s"
Day 5	15 min.	7	Choose Any Building Skill
Day 5	15 min.	7	Dr. M's Multiplication Math Facts Random "2s – 10s"
Day 6	15 min.	7	Choose Any Building Skill
Day 6	15 min.	7	Dr. M's Multiplication Math Facts Random "2s – 10s"
Day 7			Enjoy Family Time and Play Time

Week 7	Time	Chapter	Handwriting Activities
Day 1	15 min.	4	Paper Crunch
Day 1	15 min.	4	Learn "a" – "f" of the alphabet
Day 2	15 min.	4	Finger Lift
Day 2	15 min.	4	Learn "g" – "l" of the alphabet
Day 3	15 min.	4	Paper Tear
Day 3	15 min.	4	Learn "m" – "r" of the alphabet
Day 4	15 min.	4	Clay Finger Roll
Day 4	15 min.	4	Learn "s" – "z" of the alphabet
Day 5	15 min.	4	Baton Twirl
Day 5	15 min.	4	Write alphabet "a" – "z"
Day 6	15 min.	4	Card Shuffle
Day 6	15 min.	4	Write alphabet "a" – "z"
Day 7			Enjoy Family Time and Play Time

Week 8	Time	Chapter	Composition Activities
Day 1	15 min.	6	Visual/Verbal Description
Day 1	15 min.	6	Write one sentence
Day 2	15 min.	6	Story Telling
Day 2	15 min.	6	Write one paragraph
Day 3	15 min.	6	Using Full Sentences
Day 3	15 min.	6	Write sentences about an unknown subject
Day 4	15 min.	6	Describing Objects
Day 4	15 min.	6	Write paragraphs about an unknown subject
Day 5	15 min.	6	Describing An Activity
Day 5	15 min.	6	Write a one page personal story
Day 6	15 min.	6	Add adjectives & adverbs to sentences for more interest
Day 6	15 min.	6	Visual/Verbal Description
Day 7			Enjoy Family Time and Play Time

Week 9	Time	Chapter	Composition Activities
Day 1	15 min.	6	Tell a scary story
Day 1	15 min.	6	Rewrite interesting sentences, making them scary
Day 2	15 min.	6	Tell a funny story
Day 2	15 min.	6	Rewrite interesting sentences, making them funny
Day 3	15 min.	6	Tell a descriptive scary story
Day 3	15 min.	6	Write a scary paragraph
Day 4	15 min.	6	Tell a descriptive funny story
Day 4	15 min.	6	Write a funny paragraph
Day 5	20 min.	6	Begin a journal
Day 6	20 min.	6	Write a short story
Day 7			Enjoy Family Time and Play Time

Week 10	Time	Chapter	Composition Activities
Day 1	15 min.	8	This/That Confusion Technique
Day 1	15 min.	8	Word Recognition
Day 2	15 min.	8	Pre-Selected Words
Day 2	15 min.	8	Word Recognition
Day 3	15 min.	8	Pre-Ask Questions
Day 3	15 min.	8	Word Recognition
Day 4	15 min.	8	Read Upside Down
Day 4	15 min.	8	Word Recognition
Day 5	15 min.	8	Composing Sentences
Day 6	15 min.	8	Silent Reading
Day 7			Enjoy Family Time and Play Time

Week 11	Time	Chapter	Composition Activities
Day 1	15 min.	8	This/That Confusion Technique
Day 1	15 min.	8	Silent Reading
Day 2	15 min.	8	Pre-Selected Words
Day 2	15 min.	8	Silent Reading
Day 3	15 min.	8	Pre-Ask Questions
Day 3	15 min.	8	Silent Reading
Day 4	15 min.	8	Expressive Reading
Day 4	15 min.	8	Silent Reading
Day 5	15 min.	8	Expressive Reading
Day 6	15 min.	8	Silent Reading
Day 7			Enjoy Family Time and Play Time

Week 12	Time	Chapter	All Subjects
Day 1	15 min.	4	Paper Crunch
Day 1	15 min.	4	Write alphabet "a" – "z"
Day 2	30 min.	5	MONTECALVO Spelling Technique
Day 3	15 min.	6	Describe an Activity
Day 3	15 min.	6	Write in Journal
Day 4	15 min.	7	Any Building Skill
Day 4	15 min.	7	Dr. M's Multiplication Math Facts Random "2s – 10s"
Day 5	15 min.	8	Expressive Reading
Day 6	15 min.	8	Silent Reading
Day 7			Enjoy Family Time and Play Time

REFERENCES

1   Yasukouchi, Kira and Ishibashi, Keita. "Non-Visual Effects of the Color Temperature of Fluorescent Lamps on Physiological Aspects in Humans." *Journal of Physiological Anthropology and Applied Human Science* 24, no. 1 (January 2005): 41–43.

2   Basso, M.R. "Neurobiological Relationships Between Ambient Lighting and the Startle Response to Acoustic Stress in Humans." *International Journal of Neuroscience* 110, no. 3–4 (January 1, 2001): 147–57.

3   Havas, Magda. "Health Concerns Associated with Energy Efficient Lighting and Their Electromagnetic Emissions." *Scientific Committee on Emerging and Newly Identified Health Risks* (SCENIHR), (June 2008).

4   Colman, R. S. et al. "The Effects of Fluorescent and Incandescent Illumination upon Repetitive Behaviors in Autistic Children." *Journal of Autism and Childhood Schizophrenia* 6, no. 2 (June 1976): 157–62.

5   "Fluorescent Lighting Flicker," *Seattle Community Network*, accessed September 15, 2014, http://www.scn.org/autistics/fluorescents.html.

6   Xiaofei, Fan et al. "Abnormal Transient Pupillary Light Reflex in Individuals with Autism Spectrum Disorders." *Journal of Autism and Developmental Disorders* 39,

no. 11 (November 2009): 1499–1508, doi:10.1007/s10803-009-0767-7.

7   Mott, M. S. et al. "Illuminating the Effects of Dynamic Lighting on Student Learning." *SAGE Open* 2, no. 2 (June 1, 2012), doi:10.1177/2158244012445585.

8   Hirsch, M. "A review of Darrell Boyd Harmon's experimental results." *American Journal of Optometry* Mar 37 (1960): 121-37.

9   Baker, Mitzi. "Music Moves Brain to Pay Attention." *Stanford School of Medicine* 01 Aug. 2007. Web. 03 Apr. 2014.

10 Christ, Scott. "20 Surprising, Science-backed Health Benefits of Music." *USA Today*. Gannett, 17 Dec. 2013.

11 Janata, Petr. "The Neural Architecture of Music-Evoked Autobiographical Memories." *Cerebral Cortex* 19 #11 (2009): 2579-2594.

12 www.ChangingMinds.org/explanations/perception/gestalt/figure_ground.htm Changing Works 2002-2019.

13 Brengman, Malaika. "The Impact of Colour In The Store Environment: An Environmental Psychological Approach." Doctoral Dissertation submitted to the Faculty of Economics and Business Administration in candidacy for the degree of Doctor in Applied Economic Sciences. Nov (2002) 242-258. Publisher: Universiteit Gent.

14 Mattila, S. A. and Wirtz, J. "Congruency of Scent and Music as a Driver of In-store Evaluations and Behaviour." *Journal of Retailing* 77:2 (2001).

15 Douce, Poels, Janssens and de Backer. "Smelling the Books: The Effect of Chocolate Scent on Purchase Related Behaviour in a Bookstore." *Journal of Environmental Psychology* 36 Dec (2013): 65-69.

16 Hedge, Sakr, and Agarwal. "Thermal Effects on Office Productivity." In *Proceedings of the Human Factors and Ergonomics Society Annual Meeting,* Vol 49 #8 (2005): 823-827, and in "Linking Environmental Conditions to Productivity." *Psychological Sciences* 34 Sept (2005) Cornell University 34 759-764.

17 Benton, David and Burgess, Naomi. "The Effect of the Consumption of Water on the Memory and Attention of Children." *Appetite.* 53(1) June (2009): 143-6.

18 Benton, David. "Dehydration Influences Mood and Cognition: A Plausible Hypothesis?" *Nutrients.* 2011 May, 3(5): 555–573.

19 Jabr, Ferris. "Why Your Brain Needs More Downtime." *Scientific American Mind* Oct (2013).

20 Fuller, Lehman, Hicks, and Novick. "Bedtime Use of Technology and Associated Sleep Problems in Children." *Global Pediatric Health* 4 (2017).

21 Qiu, Wang, Singh and Lin. "Racial Disparities in Uncorrected and Undercorrected Refractive Error in the United States." *Investigative Ophthalmology & Visual Science* 55(10) 2014:6996-7005.

22 Guhl, Peter. Conversation on Facebook.

23 Kranowitz, Carol. "The Out of Sync Child. Recognizing and Coping with Sensory Processing Disorder." Penguin Books 2005: 256.

24 James, Karin. "The Role of Sensorimotor Learning in the Perception of Letter-like Forms: Tracking the causes of Neural Specialization for Letters." *Cognitive Neuropsychology* 26(1) 2009: 91-100.

25 James, Karlin H. and Engelhardt, Laura. "The Effects of Handwriting Experience on Functional Brain Development

in Pre-literate Children." *Trends in Neuroscience and Education* 1(1) 2012: 32-42.

26   Faber, Adele and Mazlish, Elaine. "How To Talk So Kids Will Listen & Listen So Kids Will Talk." Simon & Schuster, Inc. 1980.

27   Harmon, Daryll Boyd. "The Co-ordinated Classroom." Grand Rapids, MI, American Seating Company, 1951:1-7.

28   Gaser, C. and Schlaug, G. "Brain Structures Differ Between Musicians and Non-Musicians." *Journal of Neuroscience* 23(27) 2003: 9249-9245.

29   Rawlinson, Graham. "The Significance of Letter Position in Word Recognition." PhD Thesis Nottingham Univ. 1976.

30   Dubach, Isabelle. "World-First Brain Imaging Study to Understand Mind Blindness." June 25, 2018 University of New South Wales.

31   Hubel, D.H. and Wiesel, T.N. "Stereoscopic Vision in macaque monkey. Cells sensitive to binocular depth in area 18 of the macaque monkey cortex." *Nature* 225 1970:41–42.

32   Baron, Rea, and Daniels. "Effects of Indoor Lighting on the Performance of Cognitive Tasks and Interpersonal Behaviors: The Potential Mediating Role of Positive Affect." *Motivation and Emotion* 16, no.1 (March1, 1992): 1-33.

33   Kim GH, Kim HI, Paik SS, Jung SW, Kang S, Kim IB. Functional and morphological evaluation of blue light-emitting diode-induced retinal degeneration in mice. Graefes Arch Clin Exp Ophthalmol. 2016; 254(4):705–716.

34   Yasukouchi, Akira and Ishibashi, Keita. "Non-Visual Effects of the Color Temperature of Fluorescent Lamps on Physiological Aspects in Humans." *Journal of Physiological Anthropology and Applied Human Science* 24, no. 1 (January 2005): 41–43.

35   Baker, Mitzi. "Music Moves Brain to Pay Attention." Stanford School of Medicine 01 Aug. 2007. Web 03 Apr. 2014.

36   Cousins, Carrie. "Serif vs. Sans Serif Font: Is One Really Better Than the Other?" 2018 desingshack.net/articles/topography/serif-vs-serif-vs-sans-serif-font-is-one-really-better -than-the-other.

37   Riesenhuber, Maximillean. "In the brain, one area sees familiar words as pictures, another sounds out words." *Science Daily.* 9 June 2016. Georgetown University Medical Center. www.sciencedaily.com/ releases/2016/06/160609093644.htm.

38   Hiebert, Elfrieda, Reutzel, D Ray. "Revisiting Silent Reading: New Directions for Teachers and Researchers" 2010 International Reading Association, Newark, DE.

39   www.bloomberg.com/news/articles/2018-12-10/ screen-time-changes-structure-of-kids-brain-60-min-says. NIH Study Probes Impact of Heavy Screen Time on Young Brains. Lisa Lee, Dec. 9 2018 7:00 pm EST.

40   www.nimh.nif.gov/research/researchfunded- by-nimh/researchinitiatives/adolescent-brain-cognitive- development-abcd-study.shtml. Dr. Gayla Dowling, www. abcdstudy.org.

41   Kondo, Marie. "The Life-changing Magic of Tidying Up: Japanese Art of Decluttering and Organizing." 2011 Ten Speed Press, Berkeley.

42   Hellerstein, Lynn F. "See It. Say It. Do It." 2012 HiClear, Centennial, Colorado.

43   Dweck, Carol S. "Mindset: The New Psychology of Success." 2016 Ballantine Books, New York p 80-81.

ABOUT THE AUTHOR

Brenda Montecalvo, OD, FCOVD, FAAO, FCSO, is a passionate, sought-after international speaker. As a doctor of optometry, she specializes in vision therapy and coaches students of all ages on how to become successful in school. With a strong desire to change lives, Dr. Montecalvo uses her knowledge and ability to help her patients to be more efficient learners. She graduated with distinction from the Pacific University College of Optometry, and has provided primary care optometry in a successful private practice setting for over 35 years.

Dr. Montecalvo presents the Cedarville Seminars for Optometric Vision Therapy (OVT), and teaches her *Visual Secrets for School Success* to international audiences. She also lectures in the areas of Neuro-Optometric Rehabilitation (NOR), strabismus, amblyopia, OVT, prescribing of therapeutic performance lenses, preventive eye care, and Practice Management (PM).

She is a co-author of the American Optometric Association (AOA) Brain Injury Electronic Resource Manual, and has authored articles about NOR, OVT and PM.

Dr. Montecalvo is Past Chair of the AOA Vision Rehabilitation Section, and is a member of the AOA Education Committee. She is Past President of the Ohio Optometric Association, Past President of the Neuro-Optometric Rehabilitation Association (NORA), Co-Chair of the John Streff Invitational Lens Symposium, and trustee of the Vision

Leads Foundation. She has been a Clinical Associate Professor for the Western College of Optometry and for The Ohio State University College of Optometry.

Dr. Montecalvo is a Fellow of the College of Optometrists in Vision Development, Fellow of the American Academy of Optometry, Fellow of the College of Syntonic Optometry, and has achieved Skill Level II in NORA.

Dr. Montecalvo's interests include enjoying time with her three adult children, being active in her church, gardening, and operating a horse farm with her husband Anthony.

TAKE YOUR NEXT STEP

Dr. Brenda Montecalvo understands that difficulties during the learning years can lead to a lifetime of low self-esteem. She has seen how poor performance can chip away at one's self-worth. She hears individuals speak about roadblocks to achieving success, or why they can't do what they want to do. She has noticed that even after adults find success, they may carry the burden of poor performance throughout their lives.

Dr. Montecalvo truly believes that with Better Vision, people can lead Better Lives and will be able to contribute to a Better World®. She can help only a limited number of individuals by herself, but thousands can benefit from the *Visual Secrets for School Success*. That is why she is asking for your help. Learn how to share *Visual Secrets for School Success* with others, and think of the difference you could make with the ideas contained in this book!

How do you begin?

- Are your ready to **get results** and cannot wait to get started?

- Do you want to make your student's life easier?

- Do you think you may be able to help others that are struggling?

Go to www.BrendaMontecalvo.com, complete the intake form, and begin a partnership to help more students. On

Facebook, ask to join Vision Aces to connect with people who want to take action and help others benefit from the Visual Secrets.

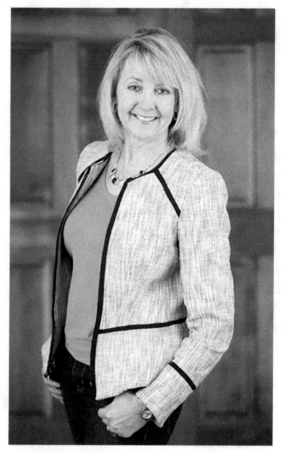

Author, Speaker, Motivational Coach

Interested in having Dr. Brenda Montecalvo work with your student, speak to your organization, or help you boost your professional success?

TAKE ACTION TODAY!

Visit www.BrendaMontecalvo.com to get connected.

CPSIA information can be obtained
at www.ICGtesting.com
Printed in the USA
BVHW041510290720
584765BV00004B/21